2/14

W9-BGF-480

LOVE ME SLENDER

HOW SMART COUPLES TEAM UP TO LOSE WEIGHT, EXERCISE MORE, AND STAY HEALTHY TOGETHER

THOMAS N. BRADBURY, PhD,
AND **BENJAMIN R. KARNEY, PhD**

A TOUCHSTONE BOOK
PUBLISHED BY SIMON & SCHUSTER

NEW YORK   LONDON   TORONTO   SYDNEY   NEW DELHI

Touchstone
A Division of Simon & Schuster, Inc.
1230 Avenue of the Americas
New York, NY 10020

First Touchstone hardcover edition February 2014

TOUCHSTONE and colophon are registered trademarks of Simon & Schuster, Inc.

For information about special discounts for bulk purchases,
please contact Simon & Schuster Special Sales at
1-866-506-1949 or business@simonandschuster.com.

The Simon & Schuster Speakers Bureau can bring authors to your
live event. For more information or to book an event, contact the
Simon & Schuster Speakers Bureau at 1-866-248-3049
or visit our website at www.simonspeakers.com.

Manufactured in the United States of America

10 9 8 7 6 5 4 3 2 1

Library of Congress Cataloging-in-Publication Data

Bradbury, Thomas N.
  Love me slender
/ Thomas N Bradbury, PhD and Benjamin R Karney, PhD
  pages cm
  "A Touchstone book."
1. Weight loss—Psychological aspects. 2. Couples—Health and hygiene. 3. Reducing
exercises. 4. Reducing diets. I. Karney, Benjamin R. II. Title.
  RM222.2.B6485 2014
  613.2'5—dc23

  2013018890

ISBN 978-1-4516-7451-4
ISBN 978-1-4516-7453-8 (ebook)

Contents

PART III
Teaming Up to Move More

A Note About Our Couples

Throughout *Love Me Slender,* you will encounter transcripts of couples discussing their health and the improvements they would like to make to their eating and exercise habits. These transcripts come from videotapes of couples who have participated in our research, and we rely heavily on them to illustrate exactly what happens in those moments when partners share their health-related goals and look to each other to make those goals a reality. The couples themselves represent a diverse group on virtually every dimension you can imagine, and we believe this diversity strengthens the general claims we are offering about how couples approach their health. However, our observations are limited in important respects: All of our couples were heterosexual, and all were young and beginning their first marriages when we studied them. This means that our samples skew, at least initially, toward healthier and happier couples. You will quickly see, however, that being young and happy does not necessarily provide immunity from health challenges and worries—in fact, health habits can undergo marked changes for the worse just as relationships stabilize, and the impending transition to parenthood often heightens concerns about health and weight. Our reliance on younger married couples also means that we have not observed important segments of the population, particularly older couples and gay and lesbian couples. Although we cannot speak with authority about the unique health-related challenges of same-sex couples, evidence does suggest that partners in same-sex and different-sex couples may not differ markedly in how they support and undermine each other's health habits.

The transcripts are accurate representations of the conversations we observed, though we have edited them for clarity, and we have cut statements that were off topic or not relevant to the point we were trying to make at that point in the text; extensive edits are marked with ellipses. Minor details in the transcripts have been changed in many instances to disguise the participants' identities. Beyond simply changing first names, we have also modified the names of particular activities and geographic locations that participants discussed, as well as names of restaurants, gyms, and diets; relationships with other people; the pet names they called each other; the slang words they used, and so forth. In our introductory descriptions of the couples themselves, as distinct from the transcripts of their conversations, we also made minor and unimportant changes to their ages, their backgrounds, their occupations, their living situations, and their family compositions.

The honesty with which our couples were willing to discuss their health-related challenges and successes inspired us to go to great lengths to disguise their identities, even to the point where we believe they will be unable to recognize themselves in these pages. All couples are unique, of course, but in conducting this research we learned that there are surprising commonalities in the emotions they experience and the ways partners attempt to engage each other in their mutual quest for better health. We have eliminated these unique features to the best of our ability, as it is the commonalities that are most important for our purposes and that we aim to convey here. We hope readers will understand that any similarity between real people and the transcripts we present in this book is random and purely coincidental.

LOVE ME SLENDER

PART I

HEALTHY RELATIONSHIPS ARE THE FOUNDATION OF HEALTHY LIVES

Part I of *Love Me Slender* makes the essential point that our closest relationships serve as the very foundation for our health. Here we explain why developing and drawing strength from the people closest to us is one of the best ways any of us can begin to make improvements in our health. But what is it about our close relationships that gives them so much power over our health and health-related behaviors? We answer this question by outlining the three basic principles that underlie our intimate relationships, and we explain how these principles can either muffle our desire for change or nurture our desire and allow it to grow stronger. Finally, we will connect the *basic principles* of relationships with the *basic skills* that smart couples use to create and support healthier habits.

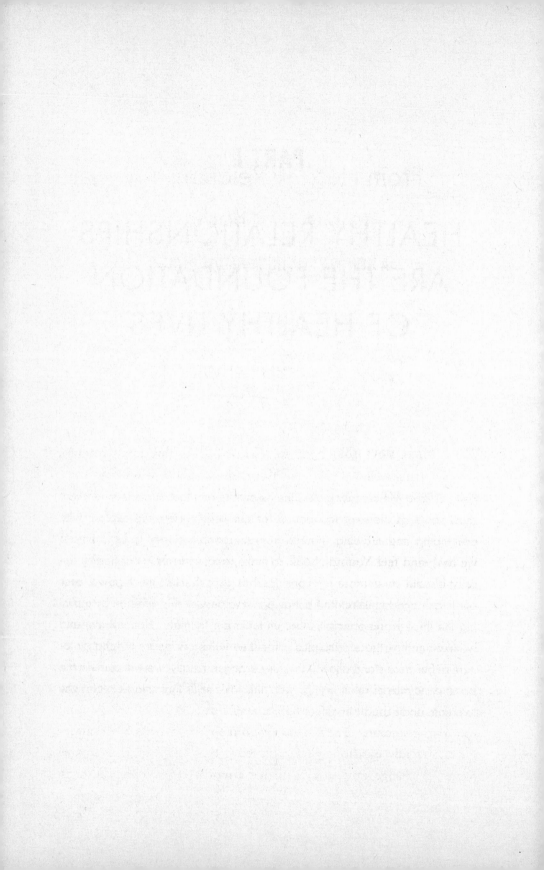

1

From Healthy Relationships to Healthy Bodies

A NEW WAY TO THINK ABOUT HEALTH

E AT RIGHT. MOVE MORE. Modern science gives us this simple formula for living well. We know that small, sustained changes to our daily routines—like eating an extra serving of fruits and vegetables at most meals; cutting down on salt, sugar, and red meat; and taking brisk walks on a regular basis—practically guarantee improvements in how we look and feel. Young or old, rich or poor, male or female, biologically blessed or genetically cursed, all of us can reap the benefits that come from the sensible habits that are known to underlie good health.

Medical professionals have been working hard to spread this simple message, and for good reason: the formula works. A healthier lifestyle *really does* reduce the overall incidence of cardiovascular disease, diabetes, stroke, and Alzheimer's disease in adults. Maintaining a healthy weight *really is* one of the best ways to prevent all kinds of cancers, second only to quitting smoking. The federal government, on the hook for covering the rapidly escalating costs of treating these diseases, is also eager for us to change our ways. With her national Let's Move campaign,

First Lady Michelle Obama aims to get us on our feet, and she tends a kitchen garden in the hopes that we will do the same. The decades-old food pyramid has been overhauled to encourage us to eat more fruits and vegetables, and fewer processed carbohydrates and proteins. Public-service ads echo these ideas, billboards tell us what to put on our plates, and the steady drumbeat of research findings, news reports, and healthy-cooking shows tells us exactly what we need to know and do to take better care of ourselves.

The message is coming through loud and clear. Many of us want exactly what the formula promises. Surveys show that we would be willing to give up shopping and watching television, our computers and cell phones, and even sex, wealth, and years of our lives in exchange for slimmer and trimmer bodies. This is more than idle chatter. In the United States, 33 percent of men and 46 percent of women are actively trying to lose weight at any given moment. We spend $60 billion a year on health clubs, diet foods, and dietary supplements in the hope of managing our weight better. We spend more than $6 billion each year on medical treatments like bariatric surgeries that reduce the size of our stomach and help us to feel fuller faster. Our commitment to weight loss and good health is genuine. We want to weigh less, we are willing to make personal sacrifices to be healthier, and we put a lot of our hard-earned cash into our fervent quest to firm up and trim down.

Yet, for all this concern and effort, Americans are no healthier, no slimmer. Some people certainly benefit from the investment, but the vast majority of us aren't getting any real traction, and the changes we want to make aren't sticking. If we are dieting now, chances are this is not our first time. Our national health is actually deteriorating and our waistlines are expanding. Two in every three Americans are currently overweight or worse, and experts at Johns Hopkins University estimate that more than 85 percent of us might be in the same state by 2030 if these trends continue.

How bad is it? Even as most people say they want better diets, caloric intake from fast-food consumption is at an all-time high, and consumption of fruits and vegetables has declined. Consider the following:

- The average American consumes twenty-two teaspoons of sugar per day, much of it through the fifty gallons of soda and other sweetened beverages that the average American drinks each year.
- 86 percent of us fail to eat the recommended two pieces of fruit and three servings of vegetables per day.
- 30 percent or more of our total daily calories come from fast food—and about half of all the money we spend on food is spent in fast-food restaurants.
- 90 percent of us consume too much salt every day.
- 80 percent of us fail to meet the recommended Physical Activity Guidelines for aerobic activity and muscle strengthening.
- 70 percent of us engage in vigorous exercise two days or fewer per week.
- 50 percent of us are almost completely sedentary.

In the end, all the government-sponsored billboards, diet pyramids, and public-service advertisements seem less like sensible calls to good health and more like lightning rods for the frustration and anxiety so many of us feel. Think about it: When was the last time you talked to someone—anyone!—who felt really terrific about his or her weight, eating habits, and general health?

Something is wrong. Having a clear, scientifically proven formula is not enough. Government warnings are not enough. Even the threats of diabetes, cancer, and early death are not enough. Somewhere between *knowing* the formula for good health and weight management and actually *being* healthy and fit, there is a huge disconnect. What will it take to fill the gap? Another diet that promises magical results? A cool app for our smartphones? Some kind of cream or supplement or boot camp? Some fancy piece of exercise equipment that promises to jiggle and shake us into shape? Unlikely. The same old methods are not getting the job done. Simply turning up the volume on the "eat right, move more" message will not work. A fundamentally different approach is required. And developing that approach requires us to ask: What are we missing? Why, in the midst of all this concern, are we failing to improve our health?

WHY CAN'T WE CHANGE?

For starters, what's missing is the recognition that *putting our desire to be healthy into practice is extremely difficult.* We live complex lives, with more stress than we care to acknowledge and less time than we need to do all the things that matter to us the most. We inhabit environments that discourage activity, reward screen time, and tempt us with inexpensive but unhealthy meals. And let's face it: we aren't perfect. We give in to the stress and the temptations. Our willpower is rock solid on January 2 but paper-thin by the time the Super Bowl rolls around a month later. Our vow to eat three square meals a day falls by the wayside as demands pile up at work, leading us to eat calorie-laden snacks in the afternoon. Our new running shoes sit idly by when our knees begin to ache or the fatigue of a long week takes its toll. Stuck in stressful lives and "obesogenic" environments, our imperfections become magnified and we easily lose sight of the good habits that we know will benefit us.

The obstacles we face in changing our unhealthy habits shouldn't come as a surprise, and neither should the dismal failure of most diets. Scholars and public-health educators have searched high and low to explain why it is so hard for us to eat right, and they provide us with several important insights. Biologically, we are not really designed for dieting. Our bodies fight back hard against rapid weight loss, responding to the threat of starvation with a barrage of cravings. From a psychological standpoint, we are not well equipped to keep a healthy lifestyle on track. We start diets and exercise programs with unrealistically high expectations, while overlooking how much self-control and discipline we will need to stay on track. To make matters worse, we consistently *under*estimate the dangers of consuming high-calorie treats like Snickers and we consistently *over*estimate the benefits of eating healthier foods like wheat bread. Sociologists and urban planners tell us that the rapid pace of modern life, coupled with the need for two wage earners in the family, saddles us with long commutes while wreaking havoc on our ability to purchase and prepare—much less enjoy—the foods we know to be good for us.

Eat right and move more? Yes, according to the latest science, improving our health requires that we abide by this simple formula. But for many of us, simply hearing the formula is not enough. *What's missing is an approach that acknowledges from the outset how hard it is for us to maintain our health. We need solutions that can be custom-built around who we are and the realities of our daily lives.* All the challenges to eating right and moving more can seem daunting. With so many forces aligned against us, we begin to think that our goals for a healthier lifestyle are unattainable. We need new strategies that enable us to take advantage of assets that already surround us, especially if they can guide us around, or through, the obstacles that we are certain to face. Making the real changes that lead to a lifetime of healthy eating and exercise requires that we develop every tool in our arsenal. But what if the "tools" we need aren't necessarily supplements, or diet books, or exercise DVDs? What if they are the *people* in our lives?

OUR HEALTH IS EMBEDDED IN OUR SOCIAL RELATIONSHIPS

What we eat, how we eat, and whether or not we exercise are all profoundly influenced by our social connections. When a stressed-out co-worker orders an unhealthy dessert after lunch, we are tempted to do the same. Conversations with a slimmed-down neighbor get us thinking about what we are cooking for dinner in our own home. Knowing that one of our friends has started to take yoga lessons might encourage us to tag along and make an entirely new set of friends—and then invite other friends to join. Seeing a brother or sister pack on the pounds can force us to take a cold, hard look at our own sedentary lifestyle. The weekly call to our aging parents cannot help but prompt us to question whether we are on the right track for a healthy retirement.

The concern expressed by scientists, government officials, media personalities, and medical professionals is valuable because it alerts us to serious repercussions of ignoring our health. (As if we didn't know already!) But it is the tremendous influence our closest social relationships have on us that fuels the consistent support and inspiration we need to *stay* on the path to well-being, and then motivates us to keep pushing forward. *Eating right and moving more—especially if we want to do these things on a regular basis and over a long span of time—are easier when we are inspired, cajoled, praised, and supported by the people who matter the most to us in our daily lives.*

Alas, most advice about dieting, fitness, and health is not packaged this way. On the contrary, doctors and fitness gurus alike assume that we enact our health behaviors in isolation, as if our relationships were purely incidental to the program. Diet and exercise books are written for individuals, as though one's friends and family members are not centrally involved—and have no stake in the outcome. Weight-loss companies and gyms, too, market almost exclusively to individuals, overlooking the possibility that someone close to us might feel threatened by the changes we are trying to make. Doctors tell each of us to eat better and exercise more, not knowing whether our coworkers or best friends will support or undermine the recommendation. Workplace wellness programs focus primarily on the employee, not on the spouse baking delicious desserts at home.

Make no mistake: there are plenty of really good diet and exercise books, fantastic weight-loss systems, great gyms, intelligent doctors, and well-crafted workplace wellness programs. We would all be wise to incorporate this information and these activities into our daily lives. But national trends indicate that these strategies are not enough, for most of us, most of the time. *Health and fitness are woven deeply and in-extricably into our intimate relationships, but nowhere is this simple, powerful fact reflected in the multibillion-dollar industry influencing our decisions about health and wellness.* It's little wonder that so many of us are not col-laborating with those around us as much as we might, or as effectively as we might, when it comes to eating the right foods and keeping our bodies moving.

A new way of thinking about health starts with the premise that coworkers, friends, and family members all affect what we eat and how much we move—and that we can't make progress until we acknowl-edge their huge influence on us. The best thing we can do to jumpstart changes to our lives is to take advantage of this influence, to use it to our benefit. But whom do we look to first?

THE ANSWER IS BY OUR SIDES

Love Me Slender is rooted in the belief that the relationships we have with other people offer us a fundamentally new set of solutions to the way we consume and burn calories. But one person in particular holds the key to the most promising solutions: your spouse or partner. Among the many people in our lives, *no one* affects our health more than our intimate partner—and *no one* in our lives can help us more. Many of us fantasize about how much better our health would be if we had a coach, a personal trainer, an on-call masseuse, and a health-conscious chef. But isn't it possible that each and every day you are waking up next to the person who is all of these things, all at once?

Millions of us have a loved one, right by our sides, who can en-courage us to make great choices about the foods we consume and the exercise we get. Our boyfriends, girlfriends, spouses, and partners have the potential to make the pursuit of health far easier than it would be without their support.

Take eating as an example. Eating right takes willpower that ebbs and flows for most of us, but our partners can give us the push that moves us past the pastries and toward the whole grains. Eating right can be discouraging, but our partner can be our cheerleader, celebrating with us when we meet our goals, and spurring us on when the numbers on the scale aren't quite what we hoped they would be. Eating right may mean giving up pleasures we dearly love (good-bye, Boston cream doughnuts!), but our partner is there to make healthy meals fun, to help us keep the menu fresh, and to distract us from temptation with their welcome presence. Eating right takes extra energy and time, but our partner can share and ease the burden of shopping, preparing, cooking, and cleaning that healthy eating sometimes requires. Think about all the ways this could work: The buffet at the Super Bowl party is mighty tempting, but our partner can remind us on the drive over about how great we have been about keeping to our New Year's resolutions. Knowing that a heavy work schedule might cause us to skip lunch and succumb to the siren song of the vending machine, our partner can slip some fresh fruit and a healthy salad into our bag in the morning. Fatigue and achy joints can derail our workout routine, but our partner senses the difference between a legitimate excuse and a lame one, and knows when to push, when to hold back, and when to offer us the Advil.

In short, what looks like an impossible task for us as individuals may be far more accessible when we team up with our closest partner.

WORKING WITH OUR PARTNERS

Deciding to take action about our health and weight necessitates changing the life we share with our partner. If our partner is hesitating to make the same changes we are, the challenges of maintaining healthier behaviors are even greater. Eating right is hard, but it's far harder with a partner who continues to buy, cook, or eat unhealthy foods—and harder still with a partner who may actually doubt or resent our desire to take better care of ourselves. If you and your partner are not teaming up to promote each other's health, then you are failing to take advantage of one of the most powerful resources you have in your lives for eating right and moving more.

Chances are good that you and your partner are already working on some challenging long-term projects together. Paying a mortgage or sharing the monthly rent? Sharing chores? Holding down jobs? Raising children? Caring for aging parents? Then you know instinctively that teaming up enables two people to achieve much more together than either can on his or her own, often with much less stress and far greater efficiency. Okay, so teaming up may not make parenting easy, exactly, but having a partner can make the task substantially easier, and that connection can make all the difference.

The same idea applies to health and fitness. When we acknowledge how difficult it can be to eat right and move more, our very next thoughts should be, *How can we team up to make this easier? If I want you to be healthy, and you want me to be healthy, how can we join forces and make sure we are pulling in the same direction? How can we work together to tailor and adapt the "eat right, move more" mantra to our unique needs, complexities, and imperfections?*

GOOD RELATIONSHIPS ARE GOOD MEDICINE

Buried deep within each of us is a hard-wired need for close connection. Psychologists call this *attachment,* and this need to bond is a potent force in our lives. When this visceral need is left unfulfilled, we feel lonely and isolated, and life's hardships fall squarely on our shoulders and ours alone. If you have seen someone in this state, or if you yourself have been in this state, then you already have a sense of what scientific literature reveals about the physical health of socially isolated people: compared with people who have solid social connections, people who feel isolated and lonely get more of their calories from high-fat foods, their hearts work harder to circulate blood throughout narrowing arteries, the quality of their sleep deteriorates, they are less inclined to engage in vigorous exercise, and their immune systems go on high alert, secreting more hormones like epinephrine and cortisol to combat the stress and inflammation that their bodies are confronting. In fact, so robust is the link between social connection and health that people with fewer and emotionally distant relationships have measurably thicker coronary arteries, and they experience more rapid progression toward heart disease, compared with people who have more support and greater social capital.

Happily, the flip side is also true. When our need for intimate connection is met, we stand a much greater chance of eating right and exercising regularly, we feel better, we are energized, we recover more quickly from disease and medical procedures, and, in the long run, our health benefits. A startling realization follows when we acknowledge the tight interconnections that exist among our relationships, our physiology, and our health. *Our weight and waistline, our cholesterol and triglyceride levels, our energy levels and our cravings—all of these, of course, are characteristics of who we are as individuals. Yet the forces that govern them are very much rooted in our intimate relationships.* Your cholesterol level is all your own, but the fact that your partner loves to eat fish certainly helps your cause. Your lung capacity is located entirely within your own body, but the fact that you and your partner love to take long walks together is certainly to your advantage. The social connection we get from our relationships can be very good medicine indeed.

But not all relationships provide the right medicine in the right dosage. Simply being in a relationship provides no guarantee that we will gain these great rewards. The health of some people is really enhanced by their relationships, but for others there are no such benefits to be had. Why might this be? First, it helps to know that two partners in a relationship tend to be highly similar to each other when it comes to their health. Coupled-up partners typically reap the same rewards, and bear the same burdens, from their relationship. Several large, nationally representative studies now show that husbands and wives are remarkably similar on various dimensions of cardiovascular health, such as their body mass index (BMI), their waist circumference, and the percent of their calories that come from fats. Even though we share no genes with our partner, health-wise each of us is far more like our partner than a person chosen at random.

Some of this similarity comes from the fact that, from the start, people choose partners who are like themselves on a number of dimensions. But for many couples, parallels in health come from the fact that, knowingly or not, they are constantly making decisions that directly affect the calories they will both consume and burn. Both partners' actions and choices create a shared environment that will make it either easier or harder for them to stay fit. When you get a new pair of walking shoes at the outlet mall, you might pick up a pair for your partner too. The family-size bag of tortilla chips that you decide to leave on the shelf at Costco can't tempt your partner when he opens the kitchen pantry. But when you bring home cupcakes from an office birthday party, you force your partner to resist the urge to nibble one. For better and for worse, then, our health and our ability to manage our health is a package deal, bundled with the health and habits of our partner.

This bundling means that when one partner improves his or her health, or lapses into bad habits, then the other partner changes in a corresponding manner. Studies are clear on this point. When one partner starts to walk more, or cuts back on sweets, or gets a flu shot, then the other partner is much more likely to do the same. And when one partner starts spending more time on the couch, drinking a bit more, or delaying the routine checkup, the mate is likely to follow suit. In one particularly dramatic illustration of this point, a study conducted over a span of three decades shows that when a husband becomes obese, his wife's chances of becoming obese increase by 44 percent; when a wife becomes obese, her husband's chances of becoming obese go up by 37 percent. Remarkably, then—and whether or not they intend it—relationship partners take on each other's health habits and characteristics— so much so that some medical professionals now recommend screening the healthy, symptom-free partner whenever that person's mate suffers a major illness like heart disease or cancer.

BETTING ON SOCIAL SUPPORT

If relationships are good medicine, what is the active ingredient? What, specifically, could we be doing in our relationships to galvanize our desire to improve our health and then transform that desire into a lifetime of smart habits? A number of nutritionists, dietitians, physicians, public health officials, and psychologists are placing their bets squarely on the concept of *social support*. Whereas social relationships can take diverse forms—including friendship, marriage, committed partnerships, and parent-child relationships—social support is that quality of connection and understanding that exists between two people in a relationship. In a word, social support is *responsiveness*—social support arises when one person is responsive to the needs of another person—and psychologists believe that this responsiveness works because it conveys concern and caring, validates something significant about another person's identity or stresses and feelings, and bolsters that person's ability to deal with problems. Social support activates and fulfills the powerful need for attachment that we all have.

Defined in this way, it is easy to imagine how social support can be the active ingredient in our relationships that drives us toward better health. What's not to like? All this responsiveness to our needs sounds like a job posting for the coach-trainer-partner-chef of our dreams! Fortunately, we, along with our partners, can fulfill these roles for each other all by ourselves. Knowing little more than just the basics of good health, two partners who manage to support each other's efforts to eat right and move more stand a much greater chance of getting the eat-right move-more formula to work for them than do two partners who have not teamed up to achieve their health goals.

Volumes of excellent research justify the wager on social support. Take a look at a few examples:

- Partners observed talking to each other in warm and supportive ways *heal more quickly* from small experimentally created blister wounds, probably because supportive communication promotes secretion of peptide hormones—like oxytocin and vasopressin—that speed biological repair processes.

- Patients with serious heart problems *live longer lives* if their partners talk with them in warm, supportive tones about their health. They recover more quickly if the partner expresses how "we" are going to manage the disease and how doing so is "our" responsibility, rather than telling "you" what you need to do to get better.

- Partners in a relationship are much *more successful at encouraging exercise* if they are like-minded in their ideas and goals about exercise. When partners are different in their inclinations to exercise, their efforts to support each other fall flat.

- People who are trying to eat better are *more likely to succeed at cutting fat from their diets* twelve and even twenty-four months later if they had partners who consistently supported their efforts.

The list of studies goes on and on, but the conclusion is surprisingly uniform: pick some habit that goes along with a healthy lifestyle—quitting smoking, sticking to a diet, regular exercise, oral hygiene, self-exams, annual checkups, using sunscreen, adherence to any number of medical treatments—and chances are high that there is a study showing that simply being in a relationship and, beyond that, teaming up with a supportive partner, makes that habit, and better health, much more likely.

SUPPORT HAS BENEFITS—AND COSTS

Aiming to capitalize on the strong natural effects of supportive relationships on health, several research teams have conducted rigorous formal experiments to evaluate whether partner support affects the success of weight loss and healthy-lifestyle programs. In some instances, just as we might expect, people with involved, cooperative spouses lose more weight than partners treated alone, and they also sustain the weight loss for longer periods of time. But other studies show no differences in weight loss regardless of whether or not a partner is involved—and some studies even show that health improvements are greater when the partner is explicitly and purposefully *uninvolved* in the program. And, to deepen the mystery, men and women sometimes report different effects of partner support even within the same study. A large 2013 study by researchers from the University of Connecticut shows, for example, that one group of overweight women lost about eighteen pounds after eighteen months if they had partners supporting them, but another group of women lost only half that amount—about nine pounds—if they were on their own in the weight-loss program. Overweight men, in contrast, followed the *opposite* pattern. They tended to lose twice as much weight when they were treated alone (twenty-two pounds) as when the experiment called for their partners to be involved (about ten pounds).

When it comes to pinpointing the one key feature of our relationships that would go furthest in promoting health, mobilizing social support is a really good place to start. Study after study shows that the quality of the support exchanged by relationship partners has a potent effect on their health habits and even on the underlying physiology that sustains their health. And yet, trying to harness that power sometimes works perfectly well and at other times backfires completely. There is a mystery to be solved here, and we believe this mystery comes down to one deceptively simple question: *What are the best ways for two people to work together to support each other's health?* As informative as they were, prior studies intending to change health habits with a supportive partner failed to produce consistent benefits, because researchers did not have a complete understanding of how partners naturally boost each other's health.

THE TALE OF THE TAPE

With data we have been collecting in our studies over the past twenty years, we believe we can now offer a solution to this mystery that has direct, practical relevance to people in relationships who want to improve their health. By videotaping more than 2,000 couples having conversations in our laboratories and in their homes, we have been able to hear all the different ways partners try to improve their health, the ways they work out good solutions, and the ways they frustrate and stymie each other. We have been able to observe the rich and emotionally engaging debates couples have when discussing health and weight and, with the luxury of a well-worn rewind button, we have been able to identify the specific things people say and do that seem to throw their conversations off track. We believe that our close analysis of these intimate conversations gives us unique insights into how social support works, and fails to work, when partners turn to each other in their quest to shape up and feel better.

Our videotapes surprised us in several ways. Yes, in a good number of couples the partners really did inspire each other toward better health. Studying their conversations clued us in to exactly how they accomplished this impressive feat. But, for many couples, pursuing health effectively as a team was a challenge. Even when partners were willing and eager to manage their weight together, they found themselves unprepared for the obstacles involved in communicating effectively about diet and exercise. But we also discovered that when couples did struggle in their discussions about health, they often struggled in fairly predictably ways, over and over again. In spite of all the different kinds of relationships, the partners' different styles and personalities, and their different needs and goals, we discovered that couples tend to get stuck in the same places. We learned that we could recognize these common traps, and we began to identify a few simple, workable solutions that virtually any couple could put to use.

THE PERILS AND THE PITFALLS OF
HELPING AND BEING HELPED

In our work, we ask couples to discuss the improvements that they most wish to make in their lives. Free to choose any topic they feel comfortable discussing, more than half of these mostly young, mostly healthy people elect to talk about their desire to take better care of themselves. Some want to diet or lose weight, others want to be more active, and quite a few want to do both. A great many of them understand that being healthy requires real effort, and that they need their partner's help to sustain it. Long before arriving in our research rooms, they have discovered that these are changes they cannot make alone.

Knowing that these happy partners were eager to help each other become healthier, we expected the vast majority of their conversations to be positive, encouraging, and maybe even heartwarming. *We could not have been more wrong.* Though many couples agreed that eating right or getting in shape was a major issue in their lives, figuring out how to team up in their pursuit of these goals proved difficult for them. These young couples loved each other—they told us as much in their individual interviews and with their responses on standardized research questionnaires—and they genuinely wanted to help each other. We could see them trying. Yet many had little idea how to do so. Time after time, well-intentioned couples fell into traps that left both partners feeling criticized, defensive, misunderstood, and paradoxically less able to achieve their goals.

Why are discussions about diet and exercise in relationships so perilous? For one thing, admitting to wanting to be healthier, and turning to a partner for guidance, can make us feel a bit inadequate and vulnerable. People who are successful in every other domain of their lives can come up short when it comes to managing their appetite or getting the exercise they know they need. In conversations that are overtly about wanting to lose those extra few pounds, for example, partners are also expressing insecurity about their attractiveness and desirability, doubts about their self-esteem and willpower, fears about aging—sometimes even uncertainty about their mate's commitment to a future together. Couples who can easily resolve disputes about household chores or whether or not to have a second child can find themselves floundering as they try to articulate these emotions. Many partners talk past each other, imagining they are simply discussing their diet or fitness when they are in fact talking about (and, just as often, *failing* to talk about) fundamental issues in the relationship.

We came to believe that these ineffective conversations were one important reason why so many of our couples, despite explicit desires to lose weight and get in shape, gained weight anyway and, with each passing year, found themselves more frustrated by their eating and exercise habits. We came to believe we had discovered a unique vantage point for understanding why so many people struggle with health and fitness, and we began to interpret all the dismal national health statistics in a new light. Suspecting that real solutions to our poor health habits might well be located in our closest relationships, we dug deeper into these conversations and learned more about how they were breaking down. An example will help illustrate what we mean.

"BUT *I'M* NOT HAPPY WITH MY WEIGHT!"

Sara, a website designer, and Brian, a dentist, are typical of the couples we have observed. When they first visited our research rooms, they were in their late twenties and had been married for three months. Asked to identify something she would most like to change about herself, Sara told us that she wanted to lose weight by exercising more. After agreeing that this issue was not a source of tension within the marriage, Sara and Brian were instructed to have a private ten-minute conversation about Sara's desire to change her exercise habits, just as they would if this topic were to come up at home. Then the couple was left alone to conduct their conversation. Here's how they started:

Sara: Okay, you already know about my issue, we have talked about this issue before.

Brian: Yes, so, what's the deal?

Sara: Now, we did make some kind of resolution before where we were going to go walking together and maybe do some other things. I don't think we talked about eating habits or anything. But that resolution didn't go anywhere. I don't even think we did it even once.

Brian: Okay, here is the resolution before we even start talking about it: You make a diet for us, you feed me the diet, you will eat the diet, you talk me into going walking and maybe ten percent of the time I will go . . .

Sara: Ten percent of the time!

Brian: . . . and we will be healthy and fit in six months.

Sara sets the stage here by reminding Brian of their unsuccessful efforts to develop an exercise routine together. Brian might have responded in a number of ways: he could have joined her in reviewing what went wrong; he could have helped her generate ideas about how to implement a new plan; or he could simply have praised her for recognizing the importance of exercise to their well-being. But from the very start, Sara and Brian are heading in different directions. Before Sara can even finish describing her feelings, Brian is already ribbing her. He is not overtly hostile, and Sara even smiles at him. But Brian's sarcastic joking sends a clear message: he does not take her goals seriously. His joking continues throughout their conversation.

Sara: I know that when you get home from work and I am there, you want me to sit down and watch TV and you don't want me to leave . . . If I say I want to go for a walk, you say, "No, no, no— stay here with me and watch TV." Which makes it really hard because, I mean, it is already hard enough for me to get myself

started and say, "Okay, I am going to do it!" but then if you try to
get me *not* to do it . . . .

Brian: Why do you have to do it at such odd hours?

Sara: Well, I mean, now I'm working every day. When else am I
going to do it?

Brian: Like, the minute I get home from work you say, "Let's go for a
walk!" I don't want to go for a walk, I just got home from work.

When Sara tries to get Brian to understand that his desire to watch
television together at the end of the day is getting in the way of her
being more active, Brian does not apologize or empathize with her. He
instead turns Sara's disclosure against her, suggesting that her desire for
his support is inconvenient and even annoying when he's trying to relax
at the end of the day. Just two minutes into the conversation, Sara and
Brian are at an impasse, leading both partners to start escalating.

Sara: Maybe you don't have to try and motivate me to exercise,
but maybe if you would just cooperate with me and say "Okay,
okay, I'll get ready and go" and not draaag your feet and say,
"Unhhh . . . why do we have to go tonight? How 'bout we go
tomorrow?" I mean, that makes it so much easier for me to say,
"Okay, we can go tomorrow." It was already hard enough for me
to get myself motivated to do it in the first place, and then if you
keep putting me off, well . . . It's just defeating my purpose.

Brian: Okay. So now this problem that's supposed to be *your* problem
has turned into *my* problem.

Sara: No, I mean it's still my problem, but in our specific situation, I
guess, it's just that, you know, I need your help.

Brian: I don't want to help!

A conversation that began with Sara asking Brian to get active with
her now finds Sara accusing Brian of undermining her. She may be

right, but the accusation does not help her, leading only to a predictable defense from Brian. Accused of being uninvolved, he withdraws further and flatly declares that he has no interest in helping his wife. Sara then tries another approach, shrewdly reminding Brian that he, too, has expressed an interest in losing weight.

> **Sara:** You've also voiced your opinion that you'd like to exercise more.
>
> **Brian:** Yes.
>
> **Sara:** So by helping me out, you know, you're helping yourself out, too. I mean, remember that one walk we did go for? It wasn't bad. We had fun! We followed the path all the way around the golf course, we walked up some hills . . .
>
> **Brian:** But it took an hour and a half!
>
> **Sara:** We don't have to do that . . . We were just kind of walking and talking. It was just an extension of what we were doing on the couch. But instead of sitting on the couch we were walking.
>
> **Brian:** I got tired. I got tired and sweaty.
>
> **Sara:** Sweat's good—sweat means you're burning calories. Plus, when you exercise, you're releasing endorphins in your brain, you know, and so you are in a better mood . . .
>
> **Brian:** Okay, let's see who can decrease their body weight by fifteen percent. First one to do it gets their new dining room table [pointing to her] or a new wide-screen TV [pointing to himself].

Brian fails to appreciate how much of Sara's identity is tied to her weight, how difficult it is for her to talk about her weight—and how much she wants to be with him. He resists her reasonable requests for support, instead meeting her every suggestion of shared activities with some complaint. His final bargain, at best selfish and at worst entirely unrealistic, only reaffirms his lack of interest in his wife's health for its own sake. For her part, Sara keeps trying to get her message across, but she misses the opportunity to motivate Brian on terms he will understand. For example, she might have said, "*If losing fifteen percent of your weight would merit a TV, what would you say five percent is worth?*" As her desire to enlist Brian as an ally starts to slip away, Sara tries to refocus the discussion at the simplest possible starting point.

> **Sara:** Honey? Okay. I said that my problem was that I was not happy with my weight, and that, you know, I would like to exercise.
> **Brian:** I think your weight's fine.
> **Sara:** I know, but I am saying I'm not happy with it.
> **Brian:** So maybe you're two or three pounds more than you should be.
> **Sara:** More like five or ten pounds.

Faced with a partner eager to lose weight, many people do what Brian does: he tries to reassure Sara that he accepts her as she is. Some partners do this with more affection than Brian is able to muster, but all are inevitably surprised when their attempts at reassurance fail to have the desired effect. Sara does a good job expressing the problem with such assurances. She has never said she thought *he* was unhappy with her weight; her issue is that *she* is unhappy with her weight. When an attempt to reassure a partner meets resistance, that suggests a failure to recognize or grasp the partner's feelings. The net result is not reassurance but invalidation, to the frustration and confusion of both partners.

Sara, to her credit, does not give up, although by this point a discussion that is supposed to be focused on her needs has shifted to those of someone else.

> **Sara:** I think we need to set more realistic goals . . . .
> **Brian:** Okay, so we'll work out a diet when we get home.
> **Sara:** Okay. Well, I already know basically what to do. But you like red meat. You like . . . pizza.
> **Brian:** I like fish . . .

Sara: You like fish?! If I cook fish, you will eat it?
Brian: Sure.

Are Sara and Brian struggling to connect because they don't love each other enough? Are they simply unaware of the basic "eat less, move more" principles of healthy weight management? No. Sara and Brian are absolutely committed to each other, and they both clearly want to lose weight. They know, too, that regular exercise is essential, and they know that substituting fish for red meat is the right idea. But it is difficult to have much confidence in their ability to make these changes. Indeed, when Sara and Brian returned to our laboratory twelve months later, they were both heavier and certainly no happier with their situation.

REWRITING THE SCRIPT

We believe that conversations like this one hold the key to getting more of us to eat right, move more, and live healthier lives. Whereas discussions that cultivate support and strengthen resolve between partners have unlimited potential for encouraging each of us to be healthier, discussions that stifle the desire for change help ensure that our unhealthy habits will remain in place. And if you are anything like we are, you cannot help but read Sara and Brian's conversation and wonder about all the different ways that it might have gone differently—leaving her feeling supported, and maybe even optimistic, about getting her weight under control. What if, instead of rushing in with his hasty "*Okay, here is the resolution before we even start talking about it*" comment, Brian did nothing more than echo what Sara already said:

Yep. I remember. We had a plan to go walking, and we never
followed through.

What if, after Sara says, "*You don't have to try and motivate me . . . just cooperate with me,*" Brian merely said, "*Okay. I can't make any promises because I am just getting home from work. You know how that goes. But, I do hear what you are saying."*

And for her part, what if Sara began not by noting their prior failures but by remembering how much she appreciated one of those times in the past when they got it right:

> Whenever I think about getting back to regular exercise, I always
> come back to that one great walk we took together through the
> park. We played on the swings. Do you remember that?

All of these statements are tantalizingly close at hand for Sara and Brian. There is nothing difficult here, no rocket science, no complex interpersonal gymnastics. Exchanging statements like these may not get Sara and Brian both on their feet each and every day after work, but it would give them the shared platform they badly need for having better conversations about their health in the future.

But there are limits to cataloguing all the twists and turns that our conversations might take. Our conversations go off track in far too many ways for this approach to give us the guidance we need. And the ways that Sara and Brian slip up may have little relevance to you and your relationship. Only a simpler and more personalized approach will work. After all, we do want a solution that is memorable, tailored to our unique relationships and circumstances, and that fits seamlessly into our daily lives.

If you were to read even a few dozen more transcripts of conversations like this, however, you would soon see a simpler approach. You would think less in terms of *specific statements* that would improve partners' health habits, and more in terms of just a few *basic principles* that underlie all health-promoting partnerships. You would start to see patterns in the ways that any two partners coordinate, and fail to coordinate, their actions as they work toward their specific health goals.

We are writing *Love Me Slender* to share the basic principles that we have discovered from studying hundreds of couples talking about how to improve their health. We will introduce you to many couples like Sara and Brian, give you firsthand glimpses of their conversations, and then help you to see the principles that underlie the success and failure of their approaches. Once you know these basic principles and patterns, you will begin to see how you can apply them within your own relationship and build them into your daily routines. Knowing these principles, and the skills that follow from them, you and your partner will be able to take full advantage of the health-promoting potential that exists in the bond that you share.

KEY POINTS FROM CHAPTER 1

- "Eating right and moving more" is a scientifically proven route to better health, yet many of us are not abiding by this simple formula. For the formula to work for us on a regular basis, we need to learn new, creative ways to put it into effect.

- New solutions are most likely to be effective if they recognize how and why eating right and moving more are difficult for us. New solutions are also most likely to be adopted and sustained if they build upon the assets and resources people already have in their lives for improving their health.

- Our health and our health habits are assumed to be characteristics of who we are as individuals. Nearly all health-related advice is directed at individuals, as if each person alone controls the foods he or she eats and his or her ability to exercise regularly. However, extensive research demonstrates that our social relationships deeply affect how we consume and burn calories.

- The relationship we share with our closest partner is especially likely to influence our health habits. Relationship partners are very similar in their physical health, and they have unique opportunities to influence virtually all aspects of each other's lives. The choices and decisions that two partners make will affect each other and the environment they inhabit, the foods that are in their home, and their inclination to be active.

- Social support is the active ingredient in relationships that enables partners to be healthy and to become healthier. However, experimental studies conducted to examine the effects of partner support on health and weight loss fail about as often as they succeed. This indicates that social support is complex, that it can backfire, and that it does not come naturally when couples are discussing emotionally charged topics like health, eating, and weight loss.
- Drawing upon extensive observations of couples talking about the health-related changes they wish to make, this book introduces and illustrates the main principles that enable partners to support and improve each other's eating and exercise habits.

2

How Our Relationships Affect
Our Health

THE THREE SOURCES OF POWER IN OUR INTIMATE BONDS

NLIKE BABY BIRDS, no one chews our food for us. We bring each bite to our own mouths and swallow it ourselves. No one can exercise or sweat for us either. Our own hearts and muscles must do the pumping. So it is not immediately obvious why the actions of our loved ones so greatly affect how we eat and exercise. Yet, as we observed in chapter 1, our partners influence these behaviors profoundly. When husbands are placed on a low-fat, low-carbohydrate diet, their wives lose weight, even if they do not go on the diet themselves! How does this happen? How do relationships gain such power over our health?

Answering these questions requires us to step back and think about how our intimate relationships affect our lives more generally. Philosophers and playwrights have been pondering this issue for thousands of years, but systematic research on relationships is a relatively young science—less than half a century old. In that time thousands of studies have explored how our intimate partners shape our actions, our emotions, and the way we think about ourselves and the world.

The more we read through all that our field has learned about relationships, the more we find that a lot of these findings can be boiled down to a small set of general *principles*. Of course, research uncovers tremendous complexity too—we are talking about unraveling mysteries of love and human connection, after all—and we certainly recognize that every relationship is unique. But, on the whole, relationships tend to follow some very distinct patterns. In fact, three principles form the foundation for the rest of this book.

What gives relationships their power? Just three things:

The Principle of Mutual Influence	Your relationship is powerful because you and your partner inevitably and mutually affect each other's thoughts, feelings, and behaviors.
The Principle of Mutual Understanding	Your relationship is powerful because you and your partner have tremendous potential to understand—and misunderstand—each other's needs, goals, and experiences.
The Principle of Long-Term Commitment	Your relationship is powerful because being committed to someone changes the way you behave and allows you to forgo short-term rewards for long-term goals.

Illustrating how these three principles operate takes us a long way toward developing specific, practical ways to support rather than sabotage each other's health-related goals. In this chapter we will discuss each principle, what makes it true, and how each one helps to explain the ties between our relationships and our health.

THE PRINCIPLE OF MUTUAL INFLUENCE

Your relationship is powerful because you and your partner inevitably and mutually affect each other's thoughts, feelings, and behaviors.

From daily decisions about how we spend our time to major decisions about our careers and children, the presence of our partners shapes the course of our lives. When it comes to health, our influence on each other seems especially obvious. We graciously accept or angrily reject advice about eating right, comfort or criticize each other when facing temptation, and give or withhold approval to spend money on gym memberships, comfortable walking shoes, or organic produce.

But the Principle of Mutual Influence reflects a deeper truth: our influence on each other is the defining feature of any intimate relationship. In other words, the influence that partners have on each other *is* the relationship. Consider this: What's the difference between you and your partner on one hand, and you and the prince of Monaco on the other? The difference is that you and your partner influence each other. The way you behave and the choices you make change your partner's experience, and your partner's behaviors and choices change your experience. This is probably not true between you and the prince of Monaco. You may know about the prince of Monaco, you may google him and decide if you like him or don't like him, but (unless you happen to know him) you cannot affect him, and that is why you do not have a relationship with the prince of Monaco. To be in a relationship is to influence someone; to influence someone is to be in a relationship with that person.

Of course, we have relationships with lots of different people in our lives, and all of them affect us in one way or another. But the influence between intimate partners is special. Specifically, influence within an intimate relationship is:

Powerful

Irreplaceable

Inevitable

The influence between partners is *powerful*. We do not just affect our partners—we affect our partners *a lot*. As we already noted in chapter 1, relationships are strongly tied to our overall emotional well-being. The quality of the relationships we have with our intimate partners is not just a good predictor of whether or not we are satisfied with our lives, it is the *best* predictor that has been found—better than our physical health, better than how much money we have, better than how much we like our jobs. This is the punch line of virtually every book about how to live a happy life. Go ahead and be a rich, successful, and famous person if you can; without the connection that comes from a good relationship, it will still be hard to be a happy person. And if you are in a good relationship, many problems and stressors lose some of their sting.

We should not be surprised by the idea that relationships affect us so strongly: human beings could not survive without the ability to form close emotional ties. Like other primates, we are born completely helpless, unable even to find food. The only way to survive infancy is through the love and care of adults, so our brains should have evolved an acute sensitivity to intimacy and closeness—and modern research suggests that this is indeed the case.

In one recent study, for example, wives were each placed in an MRI scanner and told that they would be receiving a series of small but painful electric shocks. The goal of the study was to observe how the wives' brains reacted to threat when they knew a shock was coming. The effects of anticipated shocks on brain activation were examined under three conditions:

1. When wives were alone in the scanner, their brains registered a lot of activation the moment they were told to anticipate a shock, as you might imagine.
2. When these same wives were allowed to hold their husband's hand while they were in the scanner, their brains reacted far less to the threat of the shock. Moreover, the happier they were with their marriages, the greater the reduction in brain activation. Think of that: simply holding their husband's hand changed the way their neurons fired in the face of a threat.
3. Finally, the wives were also exposed to the threat while holding the hand of a male research assistant whom they had never met

before. Did the human contact help these wives the way contact with their husbands did? No. The brains of these wives looked the same as they did when they faced the threat alone.

The influence between intimate partners turns out to be *irreplaceable*. We may have close friends whom we love and family who care for and guide us, and make no mistake—these relationships are important. Still, we reserve our greatest joys and our deepest fears for our intimate partners. Our spouses, boyfriends, girlfriends, and lovers affect us, and we affect them, in ways that no one else can match.

It will not surprise you to learn that couples facing a major transition, like a new child or moving to a new city, are happier when they can confide in each other about their hopes and concerns. But it may surprise you to learn that, for couples who feel close to each other, having family and friends outside the marriage to confide in makes no additional difference to their well-being. A close bond with your partner takes you very far down the path of good mental and emotional health. And the reverse is also true: for couples who cannot rely on each other, even those with plenty of family and friends are still at greater risk for feeling depressed.

There is a dark side to the unique influence of our intimate relationships. Just as our relationships can bring out the best in us, they have a unique power to bring out the worst as well. Ask yourself this: To whom did you tell the worst lie you ever told, and who told the worst lie to you? When researchers posed these questions to a wide range of people, they got the same answer to both: the greatest betrayals occur between partners in intimate relationships. Partners in unhappy relationships can be perfectly cordial and friendly when talking to strangers, even as they squabble with each other. The reasons are clear: we spend more time with our partners than with anyone else, we share more with them, and we reserve for our partners parts of ourselves that we generally do not share with anyone else. So our intimate partners affect us in ways that the other people in our lives cannot, for good and for bad.

If all of this is true, then finally—and perhaps this is most important—the influence between partners must be *inevitable*. Affecting and being affected by our partners is not something we choose to do or not to do. When there is someone we live with, sleep with, and wake up with, that person cannot avoid affecting us, and we cannot avoid affecting that person with every choice we make, whether we want to or not.

Examples are plenty. Consider Paul and Lisa, a dual-income married couple, both in their thirties and both with demanding jobs. Paul works as an insurance agent, and at the end of a particularly brutal day at the office, he returns home exhausted and irritable. All he wants to do is eat dinner, turn on a ball game, and be left alone for a while. Is this Lisa's problem? Of course it is! Paul may not be thinking about his effects on Lisa, but her experience that night is totally changed by having a tired and withdrawn partner instead of an active and engaged one. Lisa may well empathize with Paul and the strain of his job. She may understand what he is going through at work and willingly grant him a little space to collect himself. Nevertheless, these are emotions that *his* experiences require her to feel, thoughts that *his* choices require her to think. Each partner's experiences—even events taking place outside the home—inevitably cross over to affect the other partner's experiences within the home.

How Mutual Influence Affects Health

The Principle of Mutual Influence recognizes that partners in an intimate relationship affect each other strongly, uniquely, and unavoidably. What does this mean for your weight and physical fitness? It means that, if you are in a relationship, trying to change your health by yourself is a losing battle. If you have a partner, you are intricately tied into your partner's life and the choices your partner makes, just as your partner is tied into the choices you make.

Most obviously, our romantic partners can exert direct pressure on us to take care of our health. When it comes to eating, this pressure often reveals itself as early as the first dinner date. Food preferences are high on the list of things we consider when choosing potential romantic partners (*"Oh, so you're a vegetarian?"*). Explicit disagreements about food are especially common in the beginning stages of relationships, as couples negotiate the kinds of meals they will share together. From monitoring unhealthy eating (*"Wow! You sure seem to like those cupcakes!"*), to influencing choices (*"How about we skip the steak tonight and share a salad?"*), to outright restrictions on certain foods (*"No, you cannot have any more ice cream!"*), partners have a constant impact on each other's dietary habits.

The same goes for exercise. A big factor in determining how active a couple is going to be is whether or not their shared interests include physical activities. A couple brought together by their mutual love of hiking is likely to be a lot more active than a couple brought together by their mutual love of television comedies from the 1970s. Even if partners do not share exactly the same interest in physical activities, one can serve as trainer and coach for the other (*"Hey, let's go for a hike/run/ walk around the block!"*).

What's less obvious is that, even if partners don't want to regulate each other's health behaviors, they still do. When it comes to being healthy, the environment matters. In a close intimate relationship—and especially when a couple shares a kitchen, a bedroom, and a living room—each partner has a powerful influence on the environment they share, making certain foods easier or harder to find, and making certain activities easier or harder to do. If your partner is addicted to Oreo cookies, then you will live in a house that regularly contains Oreos. If your partner is into biking, then your home is more likely to have bikes in it, as well as helmets, a bicycle pump, and all of the other things that make it easier to go for a ride when you get the inclination to do so. When we buy food and bring it into our homes, or when we choose some hobbies and avoid others, we may think that we are making choices only for ourselves. In fact, we are directly affecting the range of choices available to our partners as well.

What's more is that just by taking care of their own health around us, our partners give us cues about how much to eat, how much to exercise, and when to stop. For example, it would be convenient if we ate when we were hungry and stopped eating when we were full. However, psychologist Brian Wansink and his colleagues at Cornell University have shown that this is not how people operate. Most of us are pretty bad at determining for ourselves how much food is enough. Our bellies don't send us powerful signals until we are either really hungry or totally stuffed. In between those extremes, we rely on how much the people around us are eating to decide what amount of eating is appropriate. Sharing a meal with a family of big eaters? We tend to eat more than normal as well. Out to lunch with a group of picky vegans? Their restraint inspires us to hold back too. Imagine what this means if you are trying to keep to a diet and your partner is not! You might want to eat less than you used to, but for people in relationships "less" gets defined as "less than my partner." If your partner is still pigging out, then "less" may still be overeating. Unfortunately, people who are already having trouble watching what they eat are especially susceptible to this effect.

Physical activity works the same way. Psychologists have known for more than a hundred years that people exercise harder when they work out with others than when they are exercising alone. If you have ever compared the experience of watching an aerobics DVD in your home with taking an aerobics class, you will understand why. Alone in your living room, no one will see if you slow down or take that shortcut. The mere presence of another person, or a roomful of other people, makes us accountable to an audience, and we tend to work harder as a result. Researchers at the University of California in Santa Barbara documented this reaction by observing joggers as they huffed and puffed past a small hill on the campus. Sometimes the hill was empty, and sometimes there was another person on the hill. When the hill was empty, or when the person was seated facing away from the jogging path, the joggers jogged past the hill at a constant speed. But when this other person was facing the path watching the joggers go by, what do you think happened? When the joggers knew they were being observed, they sped up, of course! When it comes to exercise, the audience matters, and if we are in a relationship, the most important audience is made up of one: our partner.

In our studies, we have observed hundreds of couples struggling to help each other get fit and eat better, and we have paid special attention to how the Principle of Mutual Influence informs their conversations. Some couples mistakenly view the job of reaching and maintaining a healthy weight as something that each partner can take care of alone. Like sympathetic coworkers or good friends, these partners may treat each other with care and respect, and they may well offer reasonable and sincere advice. Still, their advice is offered from a distance (*"Why don't you try one of those low-fat frozen dinners?"*), with no sense of meeting the challenge as a team. These couples underestimate their impact on each other's well-being (*"How does my drinking soda affect your diet?"*). They miss opportunities to offer real support when it is most needed (*"You travel a lot, so there's not much you can do about eating right and exercising."*). By neglecting to appreciate the positive influence each partner could have, these couples make eating right and exercising more even harder than they already are, and they find themselves outmatched by even ordinary weight-related challenges.

But couples who understand the Principle of Mutual Influence recognize that they must work on their health together. They see that no one is better positioned than themselves to be the motivators, coaches, and teammates that they are each going to need if they want to stay healthy. So, they discuss keeping fit and eating right as shared goals. Their conversations are peppered with pronouns like *we, us,* and *ours.* Each partner treats the other as a collaborator, and each feels a sense of responsibility for the mate's well-being. Rather than offer tepid advice for the other to follow—*"Maybe you should keep a pair of walking shoes in your cubicle"*—these partners gain leverage from their relationship, not only making suggestions but also providing the crucial help needed to implement them.

For example, a man in one of our studies suggested to his wife,

"Most days we talk right around lunch. How about if you take a walk then instead, or you could even walk while *we talked sometimes . . ."* Anxieties about weight are met with genuine concern, partners make sacrifices for each other, and couples describe themselves as a unit (*"We don't want to end up looking like Mike and Carol, that's for sure"*). Even if the partners engage in many health-related activities on their own, they frame their quest for fitness as a joint undertaking, and they are more likely to achieve it as a result.

Accumulated over countless moments, decisions, and interactions, this mutual influence explains why relationships exert such a powerful hold on who we are and how we manage our lives and waistlines. Mutual influence is therefore a tool that couples can take up and use, or it can be the source of many of the roadblocks that keep couples from meeting their health goals. Learning how to harness the power of mutual influence is the first step partners must take in their pursuit of a healthy weight.

Ask Yourself . . .

Later in this book, we will be offering suggestions about how you and your partner can take advantage of your mutual influence to support your goals for losing and maintaining weight. For now, take a moment to think about some of the ways that you and your partner already influence each other's health habits:

Have you made any direct efforts to affect your partner's behavior around diet and exercise? Has your partner made any direct efforts to affect your behaviors? How have those efforts worked out?

How have the choices each of you make for yourselves made it harder or easier for each of you to achieve your goals for a healthy weight?

How does the presence of your partner in your life affect the way you think about your eating and exercising?

Once you have thought about these issues, you may want to discuss them with your partner.

THE PRINCIPLE OF MUTUAL UNDERSTANDING

Your relationship is powerful because you and your partner have tremendous potential to understand—and misunderstand—each other's needs, goals, and experiences.

Alas, the road to health is paved with more than good intentions. Wanting to help is great, but it's not enough. Knowing *how* to help is crucial, and that requires the second element that gives our intimate bonds their power: mutual understanding. No one has the potential to understand us as well as our spouses or partners. Who else can keep track of our food allergies, our medical histories, and the fact that stress makes us crave rum raisin ice cream? Who else is in the position to put that understanding to use? If recognizing mutual influence energizes partners to help each other, then mutual understanding gives real direction to those efforts.

Every day, we try to communicate to our partners how we are feeling and what we are thinking, so that they will know when we need them and what we need from them. This is the give-and-take that makes our closest relationships tick. But the power of understanding goes beyond making our relationships more efficient: our partners are also our most important sources of information about *ourselves*. Think of the questions that we regularly expect our partners to answer:

"Does my butt look big in these jeans?"
"Should I go up for that promotion?"
"Was I too strict with our daughter?"
"Do you love me?"

We come to know ourselves through our partners' eyes, discovering through them whether we are attractive, effective, and worthy of being loved. Our partners hold up a mirror that reflects back our own self-image, either corroborating what we see or giving us an entirely new glimpse at ourselves. When their views of us match our own, it just feels good. In fact, when husbands' and wives' opinions of each other line up with how they see themselves, they are happier with their marriages, and more likely to stay married, than when their views of each other and their views of themselves diverge. And the benefits of being understood exist even if our partners recognize the parts of us that we would rather ignore. Think about it. Which would you choose: a partner who loves you but does not know anything about you, or a partner who recognizes your limits, your failings, and even your darkest parts, but still loves you anyway? The way our partners understand us can even alter the way we understand ourselves over time, so that our perceptions gradually come to match our partners'.

Being misunderstood, however, lies at the heart of our most serious relationship problems. When couples argue or disagree, what lies beneath the surface is each partner's frustrated desire to be known and appreciated. Think of the sorts of things that couples say when they have disputes:

> *"Will you just listen for a second?"*
> *"Can't you try to see it from my perspective?"*
> *"You're not hearing me!"*
> *"You don't get it, do you?"*

This kind of language reveals that, during conflicts, partners' desire to get their way is less important than their desire to be heard—that is, to be understood.

The consequences of misunderstandings accumulate. As couples talk past each other, unable to make their true intentions known, their disagreements remain unresolved, leading to frustration and hopelessness that get in the way of understanding in subsequent conversations. In other words, when understanding goes wrong between partners, everything else goes wrong too. If influence is the defining characteristic of any relationship, then understanding might be the defining characteristic of a *satisfying* relationship—and misunderstanding is the central problem in a distressed one. You can see why: if we have high expectations of being understood by our partners, then we are proportionately disappointed when those expectations are not met.

Our second principle refers not just to understanding, but to *mutual* understanding. When we can see the world as our partner sees it, our partner's behaviors are a lot more predictable, and that helps relationships run smoothly. Our partners are happier when they feel understood, and that makes us happier, too. In fact, helping partners to spend less time trying to be understood and more time trying to understand *each other* turns out to be the central element in one of the most effective couple therapies developed to date, Integrative Behavioral Couple Therapy (IBCT). The central premise of IBCT follows from the Principle of Mutual Understanding: the more we understand our partners—where they come from and what drives them—the more we are likely to accept them as whole people, rather than focusing on the specific behaviors (like procrastinating, or burning the toast) that fall short of our ideals. Even unhappy couples improve in therapy when they begin to understand how the things about their partners that drive them crazy may be related to the very things that made their partners attractive in the first place.

How Mutual Understanding Affects Health

Mutual understanding is crucial when couples are trying to reach a difficult but important goal, like maintaining or achieving a healthy weight. If we want to get effective support with changing our diet or getting more active, we have to express our needs clearly so our partners will know what we want them to do—and what to avoid doing. If we want to offer support to a partner who is struggling with his or her weight, we have to know what we can do to be most helpful. In both cases, mutual understanding is the oil that keeps the engine of support running smoothly. Research confirms it: even among newlywed couples who say they are completely in love, those who also understand each other accurately are more effective at providing support than those who do not.

Given its importance for a well-functioning relationship, it would be nice if understanding and being understood by our partners were second nature. Unfortunately, when it comes to thinking and talking about weight, mutual understanding can be tricky, because what partners want and need from each other is not always clear.

Consider a wife who recognizes a need to change her diet and exercise habits. When she talks about it with her husband, what might she want to hear? On the one hand, feeling frustrated by her own lack of progress, she might want her husband to offer motivation and guidance to be the person *she longs to become.* Knowing through experience that she cannot reach her desired weight on her own, she might hope that he will give her a boost, either through helpful suggestions or simply through encouragement. On the other hand, she also might want her husband to reassure her that he loves her *just the way she is,* and will continue to love her no matter what. For many of us, being accepted as we are is what it means to be loved. So this wife might reach out to her husband hoping for that acceptance, wanting to hear that his love is certain even if she continues to fall short of her weight goals.

Do you see the potential for tension here? There is a delicate balance between conveying to our partners that we love and accept them completely and at the same time encouraging them to change the way they act and the way they look. In our research, we see couples wrestling with this tension all the time. In the typical case, one partner, often (but not always) the wife, says to the other: "*I think I could probably stand to lose some of the weight I gained since we got married. What do you think?*" The other partner, often (but not always) the husband, looks back with love. And then, as he opens his mouth to reply, you see his eyes widen in fear. Listen closely, and you can actually hear the wheels spinning in his mind as he reviews his options. *If I agree with her, then I'm saying she's too fat. Can't do that! But if I say she's fine the way she is, then I'm not supporting her goals. Can't do that either!* So he stares helplessly, waiting for the earth to swallow him up and save him from what seems like an intractable dilemma.

Resolving the dilemma is not impossible, just difficult. Our partners want it all: they want us to validate them, accept them, motivate them, and guide them. And we have an obligation to help our partners do these things for us—by not being afraid to express our needs clearly and by acknowledging when our partners are trying to do right by us, even when they get it wrong. Developing the right balance is what mutual understanding is all about.

Not all couples exploit the power of mutual understanding. In the couples we see, misunderstandings are all too common and derail many discussions about food and exercise. For example, having already dismissed expensive prepared diets as a solution to his wife's weight problem, one husband we observed offered a suggestion that seemed designed to address his own needs rather than hers: "*Hey, I know . . . let's get a personal trainer. That would help you and me; I could bulk up a bit and improve my endurance.*" She was miffed—there is no money for her prepared foods, yet he is willing to invest in a trainer? The wife in this couple isn't getting the mutual understanding she needs in this conversation.

In other couples, sincere expressions of pain, frustration, and helplessness are ignored or minimized—another lost opportunity for connection.

H: When I go to the gym I feel like such a loser. No matter how many times I go it seems like I cannot make progress, especially compared to all the other people I see there.

W: And on top of that it is expensive and out-of-the-way.

We are constantly struck by the difficulties that perfectly loving, well-intentioned couples encounter when they try to negotiate changes in their eating and exercise, and time and again we find costly—but correctable—misunderstandings at the heart of these difficulties.

The partners who make the effort to really listen to each other are the partners who get somewhere, instead of talking past each other. Setting aside their own agendas, partners in these relationships focus squarely and selflessly on each other's weight and health concerns. They ask smart questions that promote deeper understanding of the challenges they are facing, and this understanding motivates them to meet those challenges. One man, a high school teacher, really wanted to exercise more, but he had trouble taking time away from work. Knowing him well, his wife anticipated his resistance, saying, *"Look, I know you love those kids, but I also know you see exercise like recreation, like watching a football game or something. This is different. This is your health we're talking about."* Yes, she urged him to change his habits, but this did not prevent her from acknowledging that he is a good teacher, and her overall message was one of concern.

Although mutual influence in relationships is inevitable, mutual understanding is not. Because partners are not and never will be identical, mutual understanding will always take work, with both partners making an effort to know each other and to be known in turn. It can be a delicate dance, but couples who learn to recognize the power of mutual understanding can embrace the challenge, and are better equipped to pursue their health goals together as a result.

Ask Yourself . . .

The Principle of Mutual Understanding suggests that people have wide-ranging reasons for wanting to achieve and maintain a healthy weight, from concerns about overall wellness and appearance to wanting more energy. The kind of support that people find most helpful depends on which reasons are motivating them.

What are your reasons for wanting to achieve a healthy weight?
What are your partner's reasons?

Having a clear idea about your own and your partner's motives will help each of you to tailor your support to the other's needs.

THE PRINCIPLE OF
LONG-TERM COMMITMENT

Your relationship is powerful because being committed to someone changes the way you behave and allows you to forgo short-term rewards for long-term goals.

Some partners get this far: They recognize that changing their health habits requires them to work as a team (*Principle of Mutual Influence*) and they appreciate what the desire to change means to each of them (*Principle of Mutual Understanding*). Together, these couples are poised to make real improvements in what they eat and how they exercise.

And then what happens? For a lot of couples, even those with the best intentions, life gets in the way. An especially busy period at work leaves less time for grocery shopping and cooking, and suddenly it's take-out pizza for dinner again. And exercise? Forget it. After being up all night with a sick child, or coming home late after overtime at work, that trip to the gym is the first thing to go.

When it comes to making a serious lifestyle change, many experts say that getting started is half the battle. But sustaining the effort is the other half, and this is where sincere attempts to get healthier fall short. The other priorities in our lives clamor for immediate attention. With all the demands on our time, how can we stay on track, week in and week out, to eat right and keep active over the long term?

Couples that sustain their efforts are the ones that take advantage of *commitment*, the third element that gives our relationships their power. Commitment, as we will be discussing it in this book, is the determination to pursue a particular course of action. Considered in this way, we realize that our lives are full of countless commitments. We commit to getting the kids to school on time, to showing up for that party this Saturday, to doing laundry twice a week.

Why do we make all these commitments? We make them because we recognize that, for any goal we might set for the future, we have to make certain concessions in the present. We might run the risk of showing up late for work by committing to drop our kids off at school, but as parents we decide that it's important for our relationship to see them off every morning. We might not have the time or energy to socialize over the weekend, but we want to invest in our precious friendships. We might put off taking up a new hobby or writing that novel by doing household chores, but in the meantime, our homes are kept neat and clean—perhaps creating an environment that allows for creativity in the long run. *Commitment is the force that keeps us focused on our long-term goals even when, in the present, we might otherwise consider giving up or not caring. In the battle between the needs of the present and our goals for the future, commitment helps give the future a fighting chance.*

Nowhere is the power of commitment clearer than in our most intimate relationships. All couples who intend to stay together have made certain promises to each other—whether they are married or not. Commitment is not the act of getting married or of staying together itself, but the long-term effort we make to keep each other feeling safe, loved, and appreciated. Commitment serves the same function in our relationships as it does elsewhere in our lives: it gives us the ability to transcend the current moment in pursuit of a larger goal. No relationship, not even the best ones, is perfectly fulfilling at every moment. Sometimes our partners disappoint us, sometimes we disagree, and sometimes we find each other just plain irritating. And yet we generally do not walk out on our partners after a single annoyance, or even after a serious disagreement. Why not? Because our commitment to being with our partners in the foreseeable future helps us to keep the short-term disappointments and irritations in perspective. We put up with temporary discomforts and compromises because we anticipate the rewards of staying together over the long term.

Consider the choices you face every time you and your partner have to negotiate something. Maybe you are in the mood for Chinese food, but your partner wants Italian. Or, more significantly, maybe you are being offered a major promotion at work, but accepting it would mean spending more time away from your family. What do you choose? The option that satisfies you personally, or the option that protects the relationship? Study after study confirms that when partners are committed to their relationship, they are each more willing to forgo their own immediate satisfaction in favor of actions that benefit the long-term stability of the relationship.

One reason that commitment has such a powerful effect on our choices is that it changes how we evaluate our choices. Just how much did you want Chinese food anyway? It turns out that the appeal of Chinese food—or that promotion, or anything else for that matter—depends on whether or not we think it will threaten our relationships. In a striking demonstration of this effect, researchers asked partners in more- and less-committed relationships to imagine themselves in a computer dating situation, and then to rate the attractiveness of photographs of possible dates. Included in the set of photographs was one that had been prejudged to be highly attractive (think Abercrombie & Fitch catalog here). When partners in less-committed relationships saw that photo, they agreed with everyone else, rating it as highly attractive. But partners in more committed relationships saw things differently. When shown the same photograph, the committed partners rated it significantly *less* attractive than most other people did. Why? Because the committed partners knew that being attracted to someone outside their relationship might threaten a relationship that they valued a great deal. Thinking about all that they would lose if their current relationship ended made potential alternative partners seem less appealing. So commitment to a long-term goal helps us resist temptation by making things that would distract us from our goals less tempting.

Relationship researchers use the term *transformation of motivation* to refer to this idea that investment in a future goal changes the way we are motivated in the present, and these transformations affect our relationships right down to the way couples communicate. When our partners say something insensitive ("*Those pants are looking a little tight on you, don't you think?*"), often our immediate gut-level impulse is often to respond in kind ("*You're one to talk, chubby!*"). Indeed, studies of couples' immediate reactions to betrayal show that, in the first seconds after the hurt registers, most people do feel inclined to retaliate in some way. If the person who hurt us were someone we never planned on seeing again, there would be little reason to resist that impulse. Ever read the comments on an Internet news site? The way people react to anonymous strangers makes it clear that people who have no commitments to each other give in to that retaliatory impulse all the time, leading to escalating cycles of insult and counterinsult that rarely accomplish anything.

However, in our intimate relationships, we often resist the urge to retaliate when we feel hurt, and the couples who resist the most are the more committed couples. For the couples thinking about staying together over the long term, that initial urge to strike back holds less appeal than it does for couples with no plans for a future together.

The bottom line is that, unless we are partnered with our own clone, sustaining a long-term relationship requires sacrifice and compromise. We are always calculating trade-offs between our own needs and the needs of our partners. Commitment to a shared future changes the way we calculate these trade-offs. By keeping our eyes focused on long-term rewards, commitment empowers us to make choices now that further those goals, even if they bring us less immediate pleasure. So, just as mutual influence creates relationships, and mutual understanding makes them satisfying, long-term commitment is the foundation for relationships that *last*.

How Long-Term Commitment Affects Health

As anyone who has ever started a diet or an exercise plan knows all too well, maintaining a healthy weight also involves tensions between our short-term and long-term goals. Confronted with a choice between steamed broccoli and chocolate cake, few of us truly prefer the broccoli.

For many people, getting on the treadmill is not as immediately rewarding as curling up on the couch. But some of us muster the willpower and reach for the broccoli or step up on the treadmill anyway, because we know it is one small part of investing in a long life replete with good health and all that comes with it, including, yes, the occasional slice of chocolate cake or an evening watching TV on the couch. Taking the long view helps motivate healthy choices just as it helps motivate choices that improve relationships.

The problem is that when it comes to diet and exercise, people generally do not keep that long-term view in mind. All of the national statistics about eating right and moving more suggest one conclusion: healthy behaviors are easy to initiate but hard to maintain over time. Consider the problems that many people have with dieting. One of the interesting mysteries about dieting is why so many people are inclined to take up new diet plans, despite their own experiences of failing to maintain them in the past. You might think that people who have experienced long strings of disappointment and frustration with dieting would get discouraged and eventually give up. But in fact research shows that *just initiating* new eating habits or a new exercise regimen is very rewarding by itself. As the first few pounds drop off, we feel excited and optimistic, and those around us comment on and reinforce our initial success. When that initial excitement fades, however, so does the new behavior—and the benefits that came along with it.

When it comes to diet and exercise, keeping our long-term goals in mind is admittedly very, very hard. In our busy lives, there are too many distractions, and too many tasks that require our immediate attention. Yes, we would like to cook a healthy meal, but that project at work needs to be completed *today,* and take-out food is so much easier. Sure, those running shoes are right by the door, but the kids need to be fed, and there must be time to give them a bath afterward. The fact is that, as helpful as it would be to keep our eyes on the prize at all times, that's just not how we are wired as human beings. Our natural inclination is to keep our eyes on the fries.

From an evolutionary perspective, our difficulty with keeping long-term goals in sight is to be expected. The earliest human beings of prehistory—nearly hairless, notably lacking in fangs or claws—had little reason to indulge in long-term planning. When life is short and food is scarce, restricting what you eat has few adaptive benefits. On the contrary, when placed in front of anything remotely nutritious, our prehistoric ancestors' best strategy was to pig out! Who knew when something nutritious would come around again? And as for getting enough exercise, the constant need to search for food and avoid predators did not leave a lot of time for lounging around. On the contrary, any opportunity to relax must have been precious and highly valued.

Human society has changed considerably since the time our species developed into its current form, but human brains, alas, have not. Although many people can now go through their whole lives without knowing real hunger, and although our life spans, especially over the last century or so, have more than doubled, we are, within our skulls, still the weak, terrified hunter-gatherers we were tens of thousands of years ago. And for those hunter-gatherers, short-term thinking, not long-term thinking, ensured their survival. A result of this inheritance is that self-control remains very hard for human beings to sustain over time, especially with regard to health behaviors.

The trick to overcoming this problem is to associate our health behaviors with some other parts of our brain that are better suited for long-term thinking. That's where our relationships come in. The Principle of Long-Term Commitment highlights the fact that, in our relationships more than in most other areas of our lives, we readily adopt a long-term perspective. Whereas the future often seems distant and hard to imagine, in our relationships we think about the future naturally and frequently. Couples in love feel comfortable using words like *forever*. Newlyweds plan to stay together "till death do us part." The very idea of committing our lives to someone, of sharing a home and raising a child together, highlights our long-term goals like nothing else. This is the third reason our closest relationships play such an important role in sustaining our efforts to eat right, move more, and maintain a healthy weight. Recognizing the relationship and the healthy future we want to share with our partner makes it easier to commit to healthier choices today.

And we can make it easier for our partner to do the same. When one partner decides to make a change toward a healthier lifestyle, the other partner may not immediately share the same agenda. That can be frustrating—why, after all, would anyone actively resist moving toward health and fitness? But the fact is that husbands and wives, girlfriends and boyfriends, don't always share identical goals, even about something as basic as their health and weight. What one partner perceives as an obvious and desirable step may strike the other as unnecessary, inconvenient, even irritating. The Principle of Long-Term Commitment, however, may suggest not only an explanation for these disagreements, but also a strategy for resolving them. When couples disagree about their weight-loss goals, what they are frequently disagreeing about is how to prioritize *short-term* rewards. One partner may want to make a change today, whereas the other partner may not think a change is necessary today. But in the *long term,* most couples are indeed likely to share the same goals, with each partner hoping for a long and fruitful life together. That shared long-term goal is the lever that may move a reluctant partner to make a change. Rather than "Do what I want us to do now," the message becomes "Let's make an investment in the long-term goal that we share."

The shift from focusing on short-term rewards to focusing on long-term goals is not easy for all couples. Ten years after their first conversations about things they wanted to change in their lives, we asked some of our couples who had participated in our research to return to our labs for further discussions. Weight loss came up again, of course, but we were surprised to see that some of the couples who had excelled at mutual understanding when we had seen them last were no longer doing so well. Pounds gained during pregnancy had proved hard to shed; diets were forgotten as job demands grew; exercise plans were abandoned as backs were strained. The small jolts and ordinary obstacles dealt out by life, we learned, were enough to push even health-oriented couples off the path they had chosen for themselves.

The couples that were thriving after ten years were the ones who most clearly appreciated the Principle of Long-Term Commitment. With their hopes for the future always in sight, they refused to let day-to-day chores and hassles get in their way. One couple was already getting specific about how the wife would lose weight after their next child, knowing how she'd struggled to do so after their first child was born. When a husband injured his knee while playing basketball, his wife helped him find a nearby YMCA pool where he could swim after work. Knowing about their parents' serious health conditions, partners cajoled each other to learn about diet and exercise to reduce their own risks for cancer and heart disease. Flexible but tenacious, these partners teamed up to maintain a healthy weight, and they redoubled their efforts when barriers to doing so arose. One husband expressed this perfectly when he explained to his wife why he was motivated to try to eat better and exercise more: *"Because it's important. The longer I'm around, the longer we're together."*

Ask Yourself . . .

The Principle of Long-Term Commitment acknowledges that reaching our long-term goals usually involves making sacrifices in the present. Some questions with respect to your weight and your health are:

What are your long-term goals? How do you want to be living your life together in ten years?

What about twenty years?

What are your partner's long-term goals?

What would the two of you be willing to sacrifice today to achieve those goals?

KEY POINTS FROM CHAPTER 2

- All of our relationships have power, but none have more power than the relationships we have with our spouses, boyfriends, girlfriends, and lovers. Our closest relationships affect our behaviors, the way we think about ourselves, and our goals for the future.

- The *Principle of Mutual Influence* says that relationships are powerful because partners inevitably affect each other's thoughts, feelings, and behaviors. Partners affect each other's health directly, through explicit pressures to engage in specific behaviors and refrain from other behaviors, and indirectly, by creating environments for each other that make it easier or harder to make healthy choices. Recognizing this principle means that couples will be most successful at achieving and maintaining a healthy weight when they treat this as a shared goal and approach the task as a team.

- The *Principle of Mutual Understanding* says that relationships are powerful because partners can understand each other better, or misunderstand each other worse, than anyone else. Understanding is especially crucial when couples discuss weight, because there can be tension between our desire to tell our partners that we love and accept them, and their own desire to change the way they act and the way they look. Resolving this tension requires that partners make an effort to understand each other's needs, and also to communicate their own needs clearly.

- The *Principle of Long-Term Commitment* says that relationships are powerful because being committed to someone changes the way we behave and how we think about ourselves. Specifically, commitment helps us focus on our long-term goals, making it easier to give up short-term pleasures that might interfere with those goals. Although our brains are not generally wired for long-term thinking, our relationships naturally prompt thoughts of a long-term future. We can therefore use our commitment to a healthy future with our partners as a springboard to motivate healthier choices in the present.

3

The Basics of Helping
and Being Helped

HOW GREAT SUPPORT IS LIKE GREAT SEX

ROADBLOCKS OF ALL KINDS—dwindling motivation, chronic health conditions, stressful work schedules, family demands, tempting late-night snacks—can thwart even our best efforts to stay active and to make smart choices about the foods we eat. At times like these, no one is better positioned than our partners to give us the gentle reminders and pep talks we need to stay the course. When the chips are down (and the chip bag is open), we need our better halves to show us the better way.

Any self-help book worth its . . . well, worth its salt, advises readers to partner up and get support. Good idea, but the reason self-help books rarely go beyond this simple prescription is that requesting, providing, and receiving effective support can be surprisingly difficult. Gentle reminders can feel like nagging, pep talks can miss their mark, and well-intended comments can register as criticism. Even when both partners want nothing more than to help each other eat right and move more, they often miss opportunities to encourage the good choices that will keep them healthy. Even worse, when partners get stuck trying to help each other maintain a healthy diet or exercise routine, they can grow frustrated and turn away from each other at exactly the time when they could lean on each other the most. A partnership that might have been a tremendous asset now becomes a liability, and the pursuit of better health remains a struggle.

Taking a closer look at a typical couple can give us a glimpse into why good support—support that really keeps us on track and propels us forward to healthier habits—can be so hard to come by. Here we listen in as a woman, worried about being overweight, has asked her husband to help her to eat smaller, healthier portions.

> **H:** We're already trying to eat right.
>
> **W:** I'm trying, but I'm not doing a very good job.

So far, so good. A positive, affirming statement by the husband allows the wife to respond by voicing self-doubt. She wants his encouragement. Now he can either bolster her efforts by highlighting the "I'm trying" part, or he can expose her vulnerability by emphasizing the "I'm not doing a very good job" part.

> **H:** I know. You keep eating junk food all the time.
>
> **W:** But, oh well. I mean, that's just me, so . . . *[nervous laugh]*.

We all want an agreeable partner, but only up to a point. This man agrees with his wife's negative evaluation of herself, amplifies it, and then turns it into criticism. He is trying to be helpful by diagnosing the problem, but he has failed to grasp what his wife needs—support, not reproach. To make matters worse, he adds some detail that is certain to be inaccurate—no one really eats junk food "all the time," after all. She accepts this unflattering portrayal (*"oh, well . . . that's just me"*), probably as a way of fending off further criticism about her unhealthy eating habits. Past experiences have likely taught her that there is little to be gained from expressing her feelings on this topic. The rest of the conversation does not go much better. When she later asks, "*One day, when we're rich and have lots and lots of money, can I have a personal trainer?*" we can understand why this woman is so eager to outsource the support that she is not getting at home.

Will this man's mishandling of this one fleeting moment doom his wife to a lifetime of unhealthy snacks and sugary drinks? Probably not. Other opportunities for productive conversations will no doubt present themselves to this couple in the future, and they might rally to the cause. But real change is hard to come by when opportunities to help are consistently overlooked. Our work suggests that how partners respond in moments like this teach them about their ultimate ability or inability to be a strong team. Repeated enough times, missed opportunities can lead partners to turn away from each other, making it unlikely that they will support each other when new challenges arise. For now, these partners want to eat well together, yet neither quite grasps how they became stuck in this particular corner or how they can get out.

HOW GREAT SUPPORT IS LIKE GREAT SEX

Healthy living is far easier when two partners cooperate. But simple admonitions to "get support" and "be supportive" barely hint at how challenging this can be and how quickly support can unravel. For starters, effective support demands a fair amount of skill on the part of *both* partners. In this example, the husband's missteps are clear, but for her part, the wife could have been more specific in asking for what she needed, and much less inclined to give in when faced with criticism.

Great support is like great sex: to do it right, both partners have to be constructively engaged, focused, and "in the moment." Both partners need to be invested in each other's needs and experiences. Talking can help move the process forward, but it is not always necessary—and sometimes it can be downright distracting from what matters most. Coordination is key, disruptions are costly, and criticism can be devastating. Awkward statements like, "But, oh well. I mean, that's just me" are good signs that *supportus interruptus* has occurred. The mood shifts, satisfaction is not forthcoming, and, as we saw here, the pursuit of health-related goals loses direction. Backtracking to recapture the moment is difficult, and the next encounter needs to compensate for the mistakes made in this one.

Moments like these are an obvious sign that partners are not reaching their full potential as allies. Real progress toward healthier eating stalls until partners learn to recognize where their exchanges go off track and how they are both missing opportunities to collaborate. Connecting with a partner in the pursuit of better health seems as though it should be simple enough. If we are aiming to improve our eating habits, for example, we simply make the commitment and agree on a plan, we buy and cook the right foods, and we eat these foods in the right amounts. Easy, right? Some couples are able to do exactly this, working hard, together, to dial down the calories and dial up the workouts, reaping the benefits in due course. But time after time we see one or both partners vocalize a true desire to eat healthier, or exercise regularly, only to come up short when trying to make this part of their joint, daily routine.

WHY ARE SOME COUPLES MORE SUCCESSFUL THAN OTHERS WHEN IT COMES TO EATING RIGHT AND MOVING MORE?

So what's the difference? How is it that some couples successfully negotiate the challenges posed by eating right and moving more, while other couples get stuck in the exact same spots time and again? Are the effective couples simply more concerned, or more dedicated to a healthier lifestyle? Maybe. Being dedicated and concerned is certainly an advantage. But the couples we have studied are all plenty concerned about their health, and all of them seem reasonably motivated to eat better, move a bit more, and shed a few pounds. Yet only some of them succeed. Well, then, do the successful couples simply know more about healthy eating or about the specific exercises that burn the most calories? Unlikely. Almost any reasonable amount of exercise will get the job done, and by now all of us know the importance of eating less fat and more fruits and vegetables. Yet this knowledge is hardly enough to get these foods into our lunch bags and onto our dinner tables on a daily basis.

Our research indicates that something far more powerful is happening. *Partners in the successful couples are working harder, and more effectively, to form and sustain the partnership they need to get the upper hand over their health-related struggles.* As the strength of their partnership grows, their ability to be genuinely helpful to each other improves as well. These couples recognize and respect how difficult it can be to make lifestyle changes, and they are sensitive to the emotions involved. Partners give each other credit and praise for making small gains in exercise and smart choices in the foods they are consuming—even if that means moving up to just one serving of vegetables a day. Yes, they do know the elements of a healthy eating regimen, and yes, they do want to eat right together, but it is their ability to form a true partnership that drives them forward toward these goals. Without this, they will get stuck and eventually abandon their desire to eat right and move more. With it, they enable each other to gain control over the foods they consume and stay inspired in their quest to burn calories.

What's special about these couples is not that the partners have necessarily achieved stronger partnerships, but that they are actively and continually engaged in the process of trying to do so. They agree there are truly important problems to be solved—*Why aren't we eating better? What can we do to support each other's need for regular exercise? How can we be smarter about all this?*—and, like detectives on a TV crime case, the partners are remarkably good at asking each other the right questions, being open to a full array of possible culprits, being patient and persistent, playing off each other's strengths, and locking on to the most promising leads. Their success is not so much a result of saying the right thing at the right time as much as a reflection of having a fundamentally different approach and attitude, as a couple, to the challenge of consistently consuming healthy, nutritious food and pushing each other to burn plenty of calories.

For some couples, improving the quality of the support that they exchange in pursuit of better health might seem daunting, even elusive. However, the good news is that our research indicates that *all* couples can develop a successful strategy, provided they know how to harness the power in their relationship.

IMPLEMENTING THREE BASIC PRINCIPLES STRENGTHENS THE PARTNERSHIP

Fortunately, learning how to provide and receive good support doesn't need to be complicated. Good support and effective helping are not about knowing how to do 100 different things in precisely the right way in 100 different situations. And good support does not mean that partners have to have superhuman skills in empathy, or that they agree about everything, or that they approach their eating and exercise in the exact same way. Instead, providing and receiving good help comes down to learning just a few key ideas and then adapting these ideas over and over again to whatever situations arise. When partners are able to do this, they become real allies in the pursuit of better health.

Better still, these few key ideas are already familiar to you. These ideas spring directly from the three principles outlined in chapter 2. There you learned the three principles that enable your relationship to affect you and your health:

The Principle of Mutual Influence: Your relationship is powerful because you and your partner inevitably and mutually affect each other's thoughts, feelings, and behaviors.

The Principle of Mutual Understanding: Your relationship is powerful because you and your partner have tremendous potential to understand—and misunderstand—each other's needs, goals, and experiences.

The Principle of Long-Term Commitment: Your relationship is powerful because being committed to someone changes the way you behave and allows you to forgo short-term rewards for long-term goals.

How can these principles help us to navigate the emotions and differences of opinion that are bound to arise in our discussions about health? How can we translate the three principles into meaningful actions—actions that make it easier for us and our partners to be healthy in our daily lives? To answer these questions, and to see how the three principles of relationships lead directly to specific types of supportive actions, let's take a closer look at a couple in which the wife is struggling to get her weight back on track.

"WOULD YOU CARE IF I GOT FAT, LIKE MY MOM?"

Asked to discuss a personal concern with her husband, Jack, Tanya—a physician's assistant well versed in the basic elements of good health—has elected to talk about the unhappiness and frustration she experiences from being thirty pounds overweight. Resigned and a bit grouchy, Tanya emphasizes how much she needs to improve her exercise habits, while also commenting on some unhealthy eating habits she would like to change. She needs help getting motivated, but we quickly learn that she is particularly intent on discovering Jack's true feelings about her appearance.

> **Tanya:** So . . . do you think I'm fat?
> **Jack:** No!
> **Tanya:** Liar! Yes you do.
> **Jack:** No, I don't.

Tanya: Okay, so you don't think I'm fat, but do you think I'm overweight?

Jack: Maybe . . . a little?

Tanya: Do you think I'm chubby?

Jack: No . . .

Tanya: Do you think I'm obese?

Jack: Of course not!

Tanya: I don't want to be fat like my mom.

Jack: You won't be.

Tanya: But why have I gained so much weight?! I drink too much soda! That's what you need to help me with: to stop drinking so much soda. But whenever you drink soda I want to drink soda.

Jack: I don't think it's the soda. I drink six a day and never gain weight. But you only drink one a day . . .

Tanya: Soda can pack on some pounds. It's full of sugar, three hundred calories. You think I'm fat, don't you? Tell me what you think about my weight and what you think about my exercising.

Jack: I don't know, I think you should at least try and get into it . . .

Tanya: But . . . would you care if I got fat—like my mom?

Jack: I would be worried about you, but I wouldn't love you any less.

Tanya: Worried about me? What would you be worried about?

Jack: I don't know, when you're fatter you're not as healthy. That's how my mom was. She got big. Try to get motivated.

Tanya: *[Whining, slouching in her chair]* What am I supposed to do? I'm just not motivated . . . I'll read a magazine or watch something on TV and I'll be motivated for five minutes and then I'm ready to eat some more cookies.

Jack: See, you're not even trying!

Tanya: It's hard when you don't have anyone to do it with you. Every one of my friends who would exercise with me is way above my level. I'm not motivated yet. And I'm not satisfied with this conversation.

Jack: I'll try and help you get motivated.

Tanya: No, you won't. You come home and you're lazier than me.

Jack: That's because I'm drained after working all day.

Tanya: So, then let's get up at seven in the morning and exercise. That's what I need to do. But I know that you wouldn't do that. You always say you'll do anything and then you never do it . . .

Jack: *[Laughing]* You won't get out of bed that early!

Tanya: But if I do get up at seven in the morning to exercise you'll do it with me?

Jack: Yup.

Tanya: Every day?

Jack: Most every day.

Tanya: No matter what?

Jack: Yup.

Tanya: You're lying.

Jack: I'm not lying!

Like many people, Tanya is frustrated by being above her desired weight and perplexed by her apparent inability to do much about it. She is a bit desperate as she turns to Jack for support and, while she is willing to acknowledge that she is "a little overweight," Tanya presses Jack for reassurance that he does not find her to be fat, or obese, or chubby. Beyond that, Tanya wants help figuring out why she has gained weight and needs to know whether he is willing to step up and exercise with her. We can see the past weighing a bit on this couple—no pun intended—when Tanya accuses Jack of lying to her about his opinions, and when she says, *"You always say you'll do anything and then you never do it."* Below we explain how knowing the three principles could help this couple join forces to enable Tanya to feel just a bit more inspired to get moving.

How Can the Principle of Mutual Influence Improve our Health Habits?

The Principle of Mutual Influence has some surprising implications for how we can support our partners. Because two people in a relationship are constantly affecting each other, changes that *either* partner makes are certain to have repercussions for *both* partners. You have probably read or heard about the results of scientific studies that compare different kinds of diets— South Beach, Mediterranean, low-carbohydrate—either with each other or with some control condition in which people follow their normal diet. At least in the short term, these diets commonly do lead to weight loss. What you may not know is that the scientists who conduct these studies eventually examine how the partners of these dieting individuals fare. Even without actually participating in the formal diet program, spouses, boyfriends, and girlfriends consistently lose nearly as much weight as the primary participants themselves lose, and reliably more than partners of those in control groups. It's almost like getting two diet programs for the price of one.

A direct reflection of the Principle of Mutual Influence, this "spin-off effect"—also known as the "ripple effect" or "halo effect"—means that if either partner is taking steps to be healthier, both partners benefit. The implication is clear: good support can be as simple as seizing the initiative, noticing steps your partner is taking to becoming healthier, and then capitalizing upon and nurturing these steps. We can be *models* of better health in our relationships, and by raising the standard for good health just a little bit, we coax ourselves and our partners to move in healthier directions. Like a jet stream does for an airplane, smart support like this positions us to move ahead faster than we would on our own.

You might think that the only way to gain this benefit is for you to overhaul your diet entirely, or maybe to convince your partner to start training for an Iron Man competition. *In fact, the Principle of Mutual Influence suggests that even small changes in our daily lives can have big effects on our health habits.* This is a potent insight. Without a big windup or elaborate discussion, either partner can make small changes that dramatically increase the chances that both partners will eat right and move more. In fact, less visible changes may be more effective in promoting health than larger, more visible changes. A moment's reflection suggests why this might be the case.

SUBSTITUTE, RATHER THAN SUGGEST. Imagine two scenarios. You wake up hungry, look in the refrigerator for your usual yogurt, only to see some strange brand awaiting you. In a hurry to get to work, you eat it and off you go, noticing that it was nonfat yogurt only as you pitch out the empty container. Not your favorite, but it actually tasted pretty good and you feel a small twinge of satisfaction knowing that you did something healthier than usual.

OR

Just as you open the fridge, your loving partner hands you a spoon and says, *"Honey, can we talk? I'm concerned about your health. I've decided that we should eat only nonfat yogurt from now on. Now I know you love your usual brand, with all that fat, and I know you don't like making changes to your diet. But I'm going to have to insist on this one. We have to take care of each other!"*

The latter version at least sounds a lot more like social support than the former version does, but clearly it comes with some pretty high costs. You, the yogurt eater, eager to get to work, are subjected to a speech, accused of being rigid about your high-fat diet, and now feel obligated to help your partner improve his or her health habits. Given these costs, most of us would probably prefer a stealthier version of support. At the very most, if your partner said something like, *"Did you try that new yogurt? It was on sale. I thought it tasted pretty good,"* you could easily agree, knowing that it really makes no difference to you, and the small health benefit is surely worth the easy switch.

In short, when you are in a relationship, you are connected to another person, as if surrounded by an invisible net. The fact that you operate as a single integrated unit ensures that all changes—even small changes—will exert their effects throughout the system. Pushing this even further, the best support is often so small as to be invisible; because it comes in under our partner's defenses, such support can make healthier decisions easier and automatic. Mindful of the Principle of Mutual Influence, we begin to see the ways in which we can support healthy eating and regular exercise in our relationships. To a surprising degree, good health in relationships comes down to partners routinely facilitating good choices. And when we can make those choices effortless, the sky is the limit.

INQUIRE, RATHER THAN NAG. How might knowing this allow Jack to help Tanya? For starters, he would recognize that they are each part of a unit, and that he has a choice whether to make the pursuit of good health easier or harder for her. Recall that when Tanya said, "*I'm just not motivated . . . I'll read a magazine or watch something on TV and I'll be motivated for five minutes and then I'm ready to eat some more cookies,*" Jack replied "*See, you're not even trying!*" Tanya already knows she is not trying, and she does not benefit from being blamed for her lack of effort, even if it is true. Our work and any number of excellent studies show that criticism and nagging almost never induce better health habits. We are too vulnerable. Most of us want to feel strong rather than weak before we launch into new health habits. Jack needs to find something positive and build on it. Following our first principle, his response might be, "*Okay, so you are not motivated in general but then there are moments when you get motivated. They don't last, but still that's not nothing! I mean, what are those things that get you motivated? Can we build on these?*"

PRAISE POSITIVE BEHAVIOR, RATHER THAN POINT OUT SELF-DEFEATING ACTIONS. Jack could praise the smallest step Tanya is making to be more active. He could help her explore the things that do motivate her, and could also fend off the self-defeating response that is likely to follow. Only the partner in a close relationship is likely to have access to this brief five-minute window of inspiration—"*Well, look at you with your running shoes and water bottle!*"—and the Principle of Mutual Influence is one of the ideas that shine a light directly on that moment. But, by not realizing his great potential for influence, Jack neglects to use this principle to his advantage—much less hers. He fails to see his own possible contribution to the solution, and he reverts instead to an accusatory statement—*"See, you're not even trying!"*—that leads Tanya to say, *"I'm not satisfied with this conversation."* And it is easy to see why. Jack fails to see that he could be a positive force in Tanya's quest to lose weight.

MODEL THE BEHAVIOR YOU WANT TO SUPPORT. And Jack could do even more to help Tanya, with a little thought but not much effort. Based only on what we heard in the earlier transcript, here are some of his options:

> Jack could stop drinking soda in the house, or even having soda in the house, knowing Tanya's tendency to drink it when he does.

> Seeing Tanya reading a magazine or watching TV, Jack could ask Tanya if she wanted to join him on a quick walk around the neighborhood.

> Jack could be up at 7:00 the next day, hand Tanya her morning cup of coffee, and ask her what kind of exercise she wants to do with him.

Our main point, then, is that being mindful of a relatively simple principle—in this case the Principle of Mutual Influence—can suggest new courses of action that stand a greater chance of bringing partners closer to their health-related goals.

Using the Principle of Mutual Influence to Your Advantage

Adopting the Principle of Mutual Influence helps us to pinpoint a few very concrete ways that Tanya and Jack could team up and exchange better support. But these are just a tiny fraction of the options that are available to any of us. By examining dozens more couples, we have been able to identify several additional types of sticking points that couples often confront—as well as the smart ways they steer around these traps:

- Focus your energy on building up each other's assets and capacities. Now is a time to exploit strengths, not vulnerabilities.
- Find easy ways to make *small* changes in the areas of eating or exercise that are most important to you. Literally and figuratively, you may need to learn how to walk before you run.
- Offer effective praise. Recognize subtle but important accomplishments and use them to convince each other that even greater changes are possible.
- Take initiative on your own to eat right and move more and see how your partner responds.
- Rise above the temptation to be critical and negative, either of yourself or of each other. Even if your partner is not yet ready to join you—*especially* if your partner is not yet ready to join you—"going negative" is unlikely to serve a useful purpose.
- Find ways to support your partner's goals for better health without him or her even noticing. No one said you couldn't be a little sneaky here!

The Principle of Mutual Influence: Assess Yourselves

As you look ahead to devising new and better approaches to eating right and moving more, now is a good time to take stock of the strengths you already possess. The statements below are designed to help you evaluate how well the Principle of Mutual Influence is operating in your relationship. Either on your own or, ideally, with your partner, read each statement and then circle the number that corresponds to how often this type of exchange happens in your relationship. A key at the end of this quiz will help you to interpret your responses.

We deal with our health and our health habits with sensitivity and respect.

0	1	2
Never or Almost Never	Sometimes	Always or Almost Always

We think of ourselves as part of a team when it comes to improving our health habits.

0	1	2
Never or Almost Never	Sometimes	Always or Almost Always

We each take responsibility for our own health, even as we support each other.

0	1	2
Never or Almost Never	Sometimes	Always or Almost Always

We notice each other's efforts to become healthier.

0	1	2
Never or Almost Never	Sometimes	Always or Almost Always

We capitalize on the small steps we each take to eat right and move more.

0	1	2
Never or Almost Never	Sometimes	Always or Almost Always

We find constructive ways to shape and encourage each other's better health habits.

0	1	2
Never or Almost Never	Sometimes	Always or Almost Always

We go our own ways when it comes to the foods we eat and the meals we prepare.

2	1	0
Never or Almost Never	Sometimes	Always or Almost Always

We struggle to connect when it comes to discussions about eating and exercise.

2	**1**	**0**
Never or Almost Never	Sometimes	Always or Almost Always

We focus on each other's failures and limitations when it comes to health.

2	**1**	**0**
Never or Almost Never	Sometimes	Always or Almost Always

We depend too much on each other to promote our own health; we do not take enough initiative on our own.

2	**1**	**0**
Never or Almost Never	Sometimes	Always or Almost Always

We ignore or overlook each other's attempts to eat better food and exercise regularly.

2	**1**	**0**
Never or Almost Never	Sometimes	Always or Almost Always

We criticize or nag each other for our lack of support and our poor health habits.

2	**1**	**0**
Never or Almost Never	Sometimes	Always or Almost Always

After adding all the numbers you have circled, you will have a score that ranges from a low of 0 to a high of 24. Here is what those scores mean:

IF YOUR SCORE WAS FROM 0 TO 7: You are either not having much influence over each other's eating and exercise habits, or the influence you are exerting tends to be more negative than positive. Double back now to review the Principle of Mutual Influence and the building blocks for translating the principle into action, and help each other identify small but promising changes that you can readily make.

IF YOUR SCORE WAS FROM 8 TO 16: You are doing a good job influencing each other in a range of positive ways. At the same time, you may be undermining these positive effects with some correctable shortcomings. Begin by cutting out as many counterproductive exchanges as possible, and then work to join around the positive changes you are making.

IF YOUR SCORE WAS FROM 17 TO 24: You recognize the influence you have over each other's health habits, and you translate this influence into better support. Solidify this strong foundation even further to ensure that it extends to all the different ways you can affect each other's healthy habits.

HOW CAN THE PRINCIPLE OF MUTUAL UNDERSTANDING IMPROVE OUR HEALTH HABITS?

The Principle of Mutual Influence is powerful because it orients partners to the multitude of ways they can be supportive. But it is the Principle of Mutual Understanding that directs partners toward the high-priority targets—the emotional challenges that make the pursuit of better health difficult. Most of us can provide pretty good support when our partners are trying to choose between the stair-climber and the elliptical machine, or between salmon and chicken. But it is an entirely different matter to console a partner who desperately wants and needs to lose weight, who cannot understand why it is so arduous to do so, who is looking directly to you to lighten the burden—or who would rather not talk about it at all.

When we think about wanting to eat right, move more, and manage our weight better, we are judging ourselves—how we look, who we are, what the future holds, whether we can change, and so on. For most of us, evaluating ourselves has some emotions tied to it, especially if we have not eaten well or exercised regularly for some time. And when we open up to our partners about wanting to become healthier, we are inviting judgments about ourselves and about the meaning that food and weight hold in our relationships. There is a lot going on here! How these feelings are handled between two partners is crucial to the flow of their conversations and to their ability to support each other's healthy eating and exercise habits. When the feelings are managed well, partners strengthen their ability to help each other reach their goals. Mismanaged, these emotions bring our conversations about exercise and healthy eating to a grinding halt.

Unfortunately, emotions can be difficult to recognize in ourselves and in our partners. Emotions like those listed below are commonly expressed—and frequently misunderstood and minimized—in the conversations we have observed:

I feel *helpless* when it comes to exercising regularly.

I am really *unhappy* about the way I look in the mirror.

I hate feeling *tired* and unproductive at work.

I *doubt* whether I can really make lasting changes in the foods I eat.

I *resent* people who manage their weight with no effort at all.

I am *ashamed* about my eating binges.

I feel *inadequate* when I see all the healthy and fit people at my gym.

I am *anxious* about my health and how old I feel.

I am *worried* about how the family diet is affecting our children.

If you have a gym membership, and you fail to empathize with a partner who is reluctant to go to the gym because he feels inadequate around all the fit people there, then your support attempts might go something like this: "*Why are you so lazy? We are members of a gym that has every conceivable piece of equipment. And it's right on the way home from work!*" Or "*Why don't you care more about your health?*" Or "*How can you be so irresponsible with our money? That monthly fee is expensive, you know!*" Not helpful. But by understanding the underlying emotions, we approach the problem from a different perspective:

"Maybe we need a different kind of gym."

"Maybe we could look on eBay for a good used treadmill."

"Working out can be kind of boring. Do you think your friend Chris
   might be able to join you?"

"You used to play pickup basketball. Is that an option?"

"Are there certain hours at the gym that you think might be better for
   you? I know it gets crazy busy right around six."

Our second principle reminds us that with better understanding comes better support—and better solutions.

Let's look at an example of how bigger emotional issues can hijack an otherwise productive conversation. This man, a real estate agent, has been married to his wife, an instructor at a community college, for two years.

H: Eating right for me is hard. It's really hard.

W: It's hard. I mean I don't think it's something that you can't change. But you're right, it's really hard.

H: It feels like we have drugs in our refrigerator and drugs in our pantry. That's what it feels like, really. It feels like there is something in there that I want to do that I shouldn't do and the desire to do it is, like, overwhelming.

W: So let's get rid of that stuff . . . .

H: I know . . . but the problem is that I don't have any control over my eating. Regardless of whether there's even anything in there or not. It feels like I don't have control over it, and I want to change that but I honestly don't know how. I guess I'll have to be in therapy for my whole life *[slight laugh]*.

W: Not necessarily. There are things you can do on your own.

H: Yeah, care to reveal them to me?

W: Some of the positive affirmations, some of the reading stuff. There are lots of books that help, you know, develop insight . . . .

H: *[pauses, sighing]* I just can't put it into that framework. I mean,

maybe it's possible, but I can't do it right now. I'm not in a place
right now where I can even think about it in that way.

Having received the clear signal that her husband needs support,
this wife starts by echoing his feelings about how difficult it can be to
eat right. After she conveys her confidence in his ability to make these
changes, he expresses in no uncertain terms the "overwhelming" depth
of his cravings for food. She is engaged and motivated to help. But then
she backs away from her husband's feelings, as though they are coals
that are too hot to handle. She offers a practical solution instead: Let's
just get rid of the problem foods. After indicating that the availability
of food is not really the issue for him, he repeats his point and again
tries to impress upon her how troubled he is by these cravings. Again
she retreats from the hot coals while also offering a practical suggestion:
Read some books! She has misread his true concerns, however, and her
suggestions land far from the target. This wife is using the Principle of
Mutual Influence as the source of her many solutions when what he actually needs is understanding. Before she can be of much genuine help,
she needs to validate her husband's emotional struggle.

Is Your Partner Ready for Change?

The Principle of Mutual Understanding directs partners toward the
high-priority targets—and this wife is not hitting the target. But what
is the target here? Yes, this man is churning through some complicated
emotions, and he would benefit from having a partner who understood those on their own terms. Friction arises between them, however, because the wife fails to understand exactly where he is in the
process of change. She thinks he is ready for practical solutions and
that the emotions are incidental to his changing, but he is clearly telling her that the emotions matter and that practical solutions are premature. These partners are like gears in a car that are grinding instead
of meshing smoothly, and as a result there is no traction to be gained,
no movement to be had. To move forward, this couple, like all couples,

will benefit when the partners apply the Principle of Mutual Under-standing.

There is a more formal story to be told about the idea of change as a whole. With his influential *transtheoretical model,* University of Rhode Island psychologist James O. Prochaska identified five stages of progress toward any specified goal. One key underlying concept here is that change takes time. We don't wake up one day with a perfect diet, or eager to run full speed on the local track. We progress through stages when we change, often holding steady in one place for a long time, and maybe even backtracking to an earlier stage, before we move forward and make durable changes to our habits. Applied to eating right and moving more, these stages might look like this:

Precontemplation—Not Ready

I currently do not eat a low-fat diet and I am not thinking about
   starting.
I currently do not exercise thirty minutes a day and I am not thinking
   about starting.

Contemplation—Getting Ready

I currently do not eat a low-fat diet but I am thinking about starting.
I currently do not exercise thirty minutes a day but I am thinking about
   starting.

Preparation—Ready

I currently eat a low-fat diet but not on a regular basis.
I currently exercise thirty minutes a day but not on a regular basis.

Action

I currently eat a low-fat diet but I have begun to do so only in the last
   six months.
I currently exercise thirty minutes a day but I have begun to do so
   only in the last six months.

Maintenance

I currently eat a low-fat diet and I have done so for longer than six
months.

I currently exercise thirty minutes a day and I have done so for longer
than six months.

For the wife and husband that we just saw, the problem is that he
is in the Contemplation stage at best, where she is assuming that he is
at least in the Ready stage. Conflict is inevitable given this divergence.
Knowing that she could apply the Principle of Mutual Understanding
to these stages of change, however, would enable this woman to meet
her husband on the step where he finds himself, not on the step where
she wants him to be.

LET YOUR PARTNER HELP YOU. Revisiting Tanya and Jack gives us another
way to see how the Principle of Mutual Understanding translates directly into improved support. One of the main reasons Tanya is not satisfied with the conversation about her weight is that she is failing to do
what it takes to cultivate Jack as an ally. She blames him for this, when
in fact she is not making herself an easy person to understand or to help.

Tanya's sense of urgency and frustration seems to be having a big
impact on Jack, an impact that Tanya fails to recognize. In truth, Tanya
is not disclosing what she needs in a way that enables Jack to be of
much use to her. After she accuses Jack of being a liar, and after the rat-
a-tat quiz about whether she is—pick one!—fat, overweight, chubby,
or obese, we can imagine why Jack might feel a bit overwhelmed and
defensive. Her feelings are immobilizing him at the very time when she
could really benefit from his help. Tanya does not see this, however, and
in the midst of the barrage Jack has little opportunity to articulate how
he is feeling or how he might reach out to her and offer real support.

DITCH THE NO-WIN QUESTIONS. Questions like *"Do you think I am fat?"*
close off options and put potential allies into a tough spot, where

answering *no* implies deception and answering *yes* implies a lack of affection or sensitivity. But knowing the Principle of Mutual Understanding would enable Tanya to see that progress toward one of her most important goals is far more likely if she can disclose her own feelings and struggles and, in the process, invite Jack to stand by her side. Whereas Tanya is pushing Jack away, the Principle of Mutual Understanding reminds us that effective requests for support tend to draw the partner in.

By closing off Jack's options, Tanya not only compromises his ability to *respond* effectively to her concern, she also short-circuits his ability to *understand* her concern. And a central element in Tanya's dilemma is that she is not quite ready to make changes to her daily routine. That's understandable. In fact, many of us think about the changes we want to make long before we actually make them. Tanya wants to be healthier, she knows she needs to make changes to become healthier, and yet she has not quite reached the stage where she is ready for action. Jack cannot be of much real benefit until he understands where Tanya is in her progression toward making significant changes in her daily habits. Once he does, he will be able to provide support that is just right for Tanya: too much of a push will only convince her that her goals are unattainable (*"When I first met you, you were running every day for at least a half hour."*), whereas not enough of a push will fail to capitalize on what little motivation she does have (*"Why not wait and see how you feel? If the time is not right, the time is not right. Why force the issue?"*). Jack needs to find the middle ground, and he needs Tanya's help to locate it.

If Jack were not so occupied with dodging the strong emotions that Tanya was sending his way, how might his knowing the Principle of Mutual Understanding help him out? How might he help Tanya to see the gulf between where she is and where she wants to be? Let's replay part of their conversation with the Principle of Mutual Understanding in mind to see how it might have gone differently:

Tanya: It's hard when you don't have anyone to do it with you. Every one of my friends who would do it with me is way above my level. I'm not motivated yet. And I'm not satisfied with this conversation.

Jack: That does sound hard. I am sorry that you are not feeling satisfied with this conversation. I am. But you just said it is hard when you have to do it alone and that you are not motivated . . . yet.

Tanya: Yeah, that's what I just said.

Jack: So, I guess, here is what I need to understand better: how can I help get you from where your motivation is right now, to the point where you are pretty much motivated to work out—even if it's just once or twice a week?

Our main point is that when partners discuss their health-related challenges, knowing just a few basic principles helps them to see completely new ways to collaborate in reaching their goals. With the first principle, the idea is, "We affect each other all the time." So, new strategies come from asking questions like, *How can I take advantage of our mutual influence to help my partner?* With the second principle the idea is, "We have to understand each other if we are going to eat right and move more." To exploit this latter principle, Tanya might ask herself, *How can I help Jack understand me better here?* And Jack might ask himself, *What am I not understanding here? Where is Tanya in the process of making changes?* Or maybe, *How can I help Tanya understand herself better on this point?*

Using the Principle of Mutual Understanding to Your Advantage
By now the Principle of Mutual Understanding should be reasonably clear to you, and perhaps you can already see how implementing this principle will supersize the support you and your partner exchange. The following suggestions make it clear that mutual understanding is a great

way to gain control over the strong emotions associated with improving health habits:

- Make sure you *both* understand where you *both* are in the change process. If you and your partner are operating from very different perspectives when it comes to making changes to your eating and exercise habits, this will thwart your ability to understand each other. Being similar in your goals is not necessary for you to make effective changes; what matters most is that you understand and support each other in the process. Work to acknowledge and accept your differences, and then look for common ground so that you can move forward.

- Consider the possibility that one or both of you are not ready to make big changes yet. Respect this stage—it is part of the process, after all—and don't use it as a reason to sabotage any improvements your partner *does* want to make.

- Before devoting much time or attention to overhauling your eating and exercise habits, focus on teaming up to address other concerns you may be facing—like work-related stress, financial problems, or not having enough time together. Then use the gains you make in these areas to push you toward better eating and more exercise.

- Do your best to make sure that all the understanding is not flowing in just one direction. If you are fortunate enough to be on the receiving end of really great support and understanding, find ways to reciprocate that—not out of a sense of obligation but because you really do have something to offer your partner.

- Refrain from using criticism to motivate each other. People rarely find criticism beneficial and chances are good your partner agrees. Even one or two well-timed sarcastic remarks or pointed barbs (*"Of course you're in shape, honey . . . if you consider round a shape."*) can sink an entire raft of otherwise superb support.

- Validate each other. Lasting change is far more likely when we are feeling good and strong about ourselves than when we are feeling weak and inadequate. Having a partner who "gets us" reinforces the positive image we have of ourselves. And while our private self-affirmations help to burnish our self-image, a partner's admiration and encouragement packs a special emotional zing.

- Help each other discover your main reasons for eating right. People want to eat better to feel more energized, to have younger-looking faces, to fit into favorite clothes, to be more confident at work, to lose weight, and so on. In the course of working to understand each other, supportive partners help each other clarify their specific reasons for making diet-related sacrifices by asking good questions and providing spot-on praise.

- Empathize with the emotional challenges of eating right. Day-to-day management of our appetites and all the food-related choices we have to make can trigger strong feelings. Regulating our eating and hunger is even more trying as a consequence. Understanding partners empathize with these feelings without judging them, sympathetically reflecting our emotions back to us so that we can understand them better ourselves.

- Provide detailed accounts of past successes. After a new mom in one of our studies expressed despair over not being able to lose weight, her husband recounted how proud he was—and how happy she was—when she lost weight several years previously: "You tried Atkins, but you didn't do it that well. But then with Weight Watchers, you went to the meetings and *you did it.*" This kind of shared history in a relationship is a unique resource, and partners can bolster each other's confidence by knowing when and how to share it.

The Principle of Mutual Understanding: Assess Yourselves

As we did with the Principle of Mutual Influence, we have identified the main ways couples succeed and struggle in their efforts to support each other through our second principle, the Principle of Mutual Understanding. The specific actions associated with mutual understanding and mutual misunderstanding are listed below, and again we invite you—and your partner—to assess where you stand on both types of actions.

We know the difference between encouraging each other to improve versus pushing each other too hard to change eating and exercise habits.

0	1	2
Never or Almost Never	Sometimes	Always or Almost Always

We offer support that is tailored to each other's specific needs and goals.

0	1	2
Never or Almost Never	Sometimes	Always or Almost Always

We ask each other whether the support we are offering is helpful and how it can be improved.

0	1	2
Never or Almost Never	Sometimes	Always or Almost Always

We try to bolster each other's self-esteem in sensitive and compassionate ways.

0	1	2
Never or Almost Never	Sometimes	Always or Almost Always

We know that some times are better than others when it comes to encouraging each other to adopt healthier habits.

0	1	2
Never or Almost Never	Sometimes	Always or Almost Always

We convey respect and understanding when we discuss deeper feelings about our eating and exercise habits.

0	1	2
Never or Almost Never	Sometimes	Always or Almost Always

We are quick to offer suggestions without following up to ask whether we are being helpful.

| 2 | 1 | 0 |
| Never or Almost Never | Sometimes | Always or Almost Always |

We fail to recognize how we are two different people when it comes to the support we each need or the ways we support each other.

| 2 | 1 | 0 |
| Never or Almost Never | Sometimes | Always or Almost Always |

We tease each other, call each other names, or use hostile humor when talking about each other's eating or exercise habits.

| 2 | 1 | 0 |
| Never or Almost Never | Sometimes | Always or Almost Always |

We make it difficult to understand and support each other.

| 2 | 1 | 0 |
| Never or Almost Never | Sometimes | Always or Almost Always |

We complain about the support we receive without providing constructive suggestions for improvement.

| 2 | 1 | 0 |
| Never or Almost Never | Sometimes | Always or Almost Always |

We tend to misunderstand each other's goals and motivations for being healthier.

| 2 | 1 | 0 |
| Never or Almost Never | Sometimes | Always or Almost Always |

After adding all the numbers you have circled, you will have a score that ranges from a low of 0 to a high of 24. Here is what those scores mean:

IF YOUR SCORE WAS FROM 0 TO 7: Your inclination to understand each other around healthier eating and regular exercise is not yet as strong as it could be in your relationship. Left unaddressed, this may slow your progress toward regular exercise and a healthier diet. Your main goal now is to get to a shared understanding of what you each want and need, while recognizing that you can still be different in how you pursue better health.

IF YOUR SCORE WAS FROM 8 TO 16: You connect pretty well when it comes to eating right and moving more. At the same time, differences and misunderstandings between you might be limiting your ability to take full advantage of your relationship. Listen even more closely to what you are each saying about your unique challenges, and be clear in expressing the amount and type of support you are seeking.

IF YOUR SCORE WAS FROM 17 TO 24: You understand each other's health habits and goals quite well, and misunderstandings in this area tend to be few. This is no small accomplishment. Even still, you want to translate this understanding into real changes in your diet and your workout routine.

HOW CAN THE PRINCIPLE OF LONG-TERM COMMITMENT IMPROVE OUR HEALTH HABITS?

The first and second principles of Mutual Influence and Mutual Understanding place a premium on staying upbeat and positive. Nagging, criticism, and fault-finding all but destroy our ability to influence each other well, and blaming, complaining, and a lack of empathy can have only a toxic effect on mutual understanding. You can get pretty far in a relationship by being genuinely nice and sincere. And you will not be surprised to learn that plenty of research indicates that partners who treat each other with more kindness and less hostility tend to be in happier relationships than otherwise similar partners who treat each other badly. But a new line of research puts a completely different spin on how our relationships work.

Emerging studies clearly show that if you want to help your partner change and improve, it really helps to be open and direct—even if this comes across as being a bit negative or a tad insistent. We are not advocating character attacks, obviously, nor are we recommending that you berate your partner. But there are times—and poor health habits are likely to be one of those times—when providing clear expectations for acceptable behavior produces lasting benefits. What's interesting about this work is that it posits that tactful but toothless strategies feel good in the short term, but they do not instigate much change: "*Well, honey, if you really are twenty-five pounds overweight like you say, then maybe we shouldn't be barbecuing steak and drinking wine every weekend this summer.*" Most of us would agree with this statement and keep right on cooking. More direct and forthright tactics don't feel so great in the short term but by comparison stand a much greater chance of bringing about the change we want to see:

> I agree with your doctor that you could stand to lose a significant
> amount of weight, and I care about you too much to let these bad
> habits become the death of us. So, step one involves our cutting back
> the beef barbecues to once a month at most, using leaner cuts of
> beef, and that probably means cutting down on the baked potatoes
> too; we can barbecue chicken or fish other weekends if you want.
> Step two: I think we get one or maybe two really great bottles of
> red wine, and drink that only when we eat red meat, and we savor it,
> we make it last all summer. This must be done. I mean, I am sorry to
> have to tell you, but, you have run out of options and now is the best
> time. We can take stock and see where things are come September.

Few of us would willingly forgo the weekly grilled porterhouse and baked potato soaked with sour cream and butter. Yet the "tough love" approach that this partner displays really delivers the goods. This strategy is one of several derived from the Principle of Long-Term Commitment. Adding this third principle to our arsenal makes for a very strong and complete set of effective support strategies. Let's revisit Tanya and Jack one last time to see how knowing this principle might strengthen their conversation.

For people like Tanya, the speed bumps toward better health are all too apparent. Tanya's struggles to lose weight and get motivated have expanded beyond what she can manage by herself, and as a result she needs to draw upon whatever commitment exists between her and Jack. You have probably already noticed how Tanya and Jack are negotiating their long-term commitment rather explicitly.

> **Tanya:** So, then, let's get up at seven in the morning and exercise.
> That's what I need to do. But I know that you wouldn't do that.
> You always say you'll do anything and then you never do it . . .

Tanya is questioning Jack's commitment to helping her in this one particular arena of her life. She is in effect asking, "Are you going to be there for me? Can I trust you to hold up your end of the agreement?" And her skepticism has a sharp edge to it: she "knows" he will not get up to exercise with her at 7:00. After all, from her perspective, Jack "always" says he will do "anything" and then "never" does it. Presenting her views in this way forces Jack to dig himself out of a deep hole. Maybe Tanya says these things to lower her expectations of him, or to lessen her own disappointment, or to make Jack feel bad for having disappointed her in the past. No matter what, Jack really has little choice over how to respond. Saying *no* is not an option for Jack, given the intensity of Tanya's emotions on this subject, her willingness to paint him as the bad guy, and, more benevolently, a genuine desire on Jack's part to help his wife get moving again.

As the conversation continues, we can see that neither Tanya nor Jack fully appreciates how the Principle of Long-Term Commitment could connect them with specific actions that would serve them better.

Jack: *[laughing]* You won't get out of bed that early!

Tanya: But if I do get up at seven in the morning to exercise you'll do it with me?

Jack: Yup.

Tanya: Every day?

Jack: Most every day.

Tanya: No matter what?

Jack: Yup.

Tanya: You're lying.

Jack: I'm not lying!

At first Tanya seems to have the right idea. She senses that some of the power in the relationship comes from Jack's waking up next to her; at least in this physical sense he is there for her, very close at hand. But the conversation breaks down in several ways. First, Tanya fails to take Jack at his word when he does agree to her request, and she fails to remind him how critically important this commitment is to her. Second, she is relying heavily on him and offers little in return, not even thanks, or appreciation, or any acknowledgment that trying to motivate another person to exercise may not be the most appealing task to undertake at 7:00 a.m. Tanya is taking Jack for granted here, assuming that he is committed to her but not really respecting the value of that commitment. She is disparaging the commitment instead of using it to her advantage.

For his part, Jack misses some big opportunities to implement the Principle of Long-Term Commitment too. Take a closer look at what Jack said to Tanya after she made this request.

Tanya: Soda can pack on some pounds. It's full of sugar, three hundred calories . . . . You think I'm fat, don't you? Tell me what you think about my weight and what you think about my exercising.

Jack: I don't know, I think you should at least try and get into it . . .

Tanya has asked Jack for his opinion. Jack's response here is not un-reasonable, especially given that her request is a loaded one. But few of us would find Jack's comment helpful. How might knowing the Prin-ciple of Long-Term Commitment suggest a better approach? Here is one possibility:

Tanya: . . .You think I'm fat, don't you? Tell me what you think about my weight and what you think about my exercising.

Jack: Are you asking me my honest opinion?

Tanya: Well, yeah.

Jack: Correct me if I am wrong, but I think you are heavier now than at any other time since I have known you.

Tanya: Uh, that's right.

Jack: That's a concern for me, not because it affects my feelings for you—it never will—but because this is *your health* we are talking about. I want you to take better care of yourself, for your sake, and for our sake. And if you've gained weight at the same time you have slacked off on your exercise, well, then, to me that's a good sign you need to find a way to get moving again.

Seconds later, Jack overlooks another great opening for using this principle.

Tanya: But . . . would you care if I got fat—like my mom?

Jack: I would be worried about you but I wouldn't love you any less.

Tanya: Worried about me? What would you be worried about?

Jack: I don't know, when you're fatter you're not as healthy. That's how my mom was. She got big. Try to get motivated.

Comparing his wife to his overweight mother might not be Jack's best idea but, again, there are worse things for him to say. Even so, Tanya needs stronger medicine, and Jack needs to use the strength of their re-lationship to give his words some punch.

Tanya: Worried about me? What would you be worried about?

Jack: Worried about you?! Of course I am worried about you. You're my wife, and I want you to be healthy and happy, for goodness' sake. Our kids are going to need a healthy mom! The thing is, I am completely confident in your ability to get back on track with your exercising, because I have seen you do it before. But you need to dedicate yourself to this now. You do. I am not saying it's easy, I am just saying I know you are capable of doing it.

Eating right and moving more are genuinely hard for most of us, and it's so easy to cave when we're facing such an overwhelming task. When one person confronts this turbulence head-on—"It's hard to keep going. My regular routine is boring and I am stuck here. Can you help motivate me?"—the Principle of Long-Term Commitment can empower both partners to ride out the storm knowing that smooth sailing is on the horizon. The person seeking to make the change needs to draw upon and nurture the commitment that resides within the relationship ("*I want to get up at seven and exercise. I know it is going to be hard but I'm not sure I can get started without you. I know it is asking a lot, but I would love it if you could get up and talk me through that*"). And so does the person aiming to offer some support ("*It really is hard, and it will take time to see results. But it will be worth it. Let's start tomorrow and try to be really consistent about this*"). Limp offers of support are flimsy defenses against the strong urges we have to eat unhealthy foods and cut back on exercise, but the Principle of Long-Term Commitment is the key to bolstering our defenses and making healthier choices.

Using the Principle of Long-Term Commitment to Your Advantage

You can probably see how using the Principle of Long-Term Commitment requires some delicacy and tact, and maybe even a dash of courage, to implement well. As much as we might value the commitment we share with our partners, the "tough love" approach implied by this principle can feel unkind or insensitive. After all, some friction is built into this principle, combining as it does one message we all want to hear, *"When we think long-term, all the things we are doing now will help to keep us healthy and thriving. Isn't that great?!"* with a message that can chafe, *"In the short term, we are going to have to make some hard choices and push each other to uphold those commitments."* The key is to convey both messages clearly, and to do so in a way that reflects the unique circumstances within your relationship. With this general goal in mind, here are some specific points to consider as you work to implement this third principle into your relationship:

- Focus less on the outcome of your efforts (*"No matter what I do, my weight stays the same!"*) and more on the healthy habits themselves (*"I had yogurt with fruit every day this week—not a single bagel!"*). Use your relationship to change what you can control—healthy actions—and build consistency in that area.

- Tap into the deep values that you know you both share, and connect those values to healthier living. We have seen couples gain strength from their religious faith, their memories of a beloved relative who passed away much too soon, or their love of family and children, all as sources of inspiration. This is a big part of who you are and why you uphold your commitments, and reminding yourselves of these values can give you extra motivation for better health.

- Remember that the third principle requires careful delivery of two messages: *1) there are aspects of our relationship that give us strength, and 2) we can use that strength to remind each other to make hard short-term sacrifices knowing that long-term health benefits await us.* Talk with each other to make sure that you are both delivering both parts of the message—especially the second part—in the most effective and non-threatening ways possible.

- Shift away from shorter-term unhealthy dieting strategies to a series of small, gradual changes that are more likely to stick. This is the long view that the Principle of Long-Term Commitment can bring.

- Plan for disruptions. Many couples are able to use our third principle to eat pretty well and exercise with some regularity. But when work schedules change, when the in-laws visit, and when the holiday parties hit the calendar in December, all these good habits can slip away. In situations like these, either plan in advance to recover from going off schedule—Hello, January 1—or, better yet, partner up before the disruptions and help each other maintain good health habits as much as possible.

- Be flexible. Keep in mind that injuries can force you to adjust your workout strategy. Your weekly tennis match is great until the tendons in your forearm start to hurt, and your daily run works for you until you sprain your ankle. Even the healthiest of couples do not have complete control over their health, but they can demonstrate resilience by finding new options for exercise.

The Principle of Long-Term Commitment: Assess Yourselves

To help you clarify and evaluate your unique circumstances, we have identified a total of twelve relatively effective and ineffective ways that couples in our studies have applied the Principle of Long-Term Commitment. Either on your own or, ideally, with your partner, read each statement below and then indicate how often this happens in your relationship.

We understand that our health is a daily responsibility and a lifelong pursuit.

0	**1**	**2**
Never or Almost Never	Sometimes	Always or Almost Always

We are good at acknowledging and rewarding the short-term sacrifices we each make to achieve our longer-term health goals.

0	**1**	**2**
Never or Almost Never	Sometimes	Always or Almost Always

We help each other develop the patience and strength we need to make lasting improvements in our health habits.

0	1	2
Never or Almost Never	Sometimes	Always or Almost Always

We forgive each other for being less than perfect in the long-term pursuit of good health, while remaining steadfast in the importance of this goal.

0	1	2
Never or Almost Never	Sometimes	Always or Almost Always

We can convince each other to do the hard things needed to get healthy and stay healthy.

0	1	2
Never or Almost Never	Sometimes	Always or Almost Always

We hold each other accountable for the health-related commitments we make.

0	1	2
Never or Almost Never	Sometimes	Always or Almost Always

We treat health as an "on-again, off-again" pursuit.

2	1	0
Never or Almost Never	Sometimes	Always or Almost Always

We dwell on the short-term difficulties of eating right and moving more, without recognizing that these difficulties will eventually have longer-term benefits.

2	1	0
Never or Almost Never	Sometimes	Always or Almost Always

We often neglect or forget whatever commitments we make to maintaining our own health habits.

2	1	0
Never or Almost Never	Sometimes	Always or Almost Always

We fail to take action when either of us stops exercising or when our eating habits start to slip.

2	**1**	**0**
Never or Almost Never	Sometimes	Always or Almost Always

We fail to follow through on whatever commitments we make to supporting each other's health habits.

2	**1**	**0**
Never or Almost Never	Sometimes	Always or Almost Always

We get easily thrown off track when our health and health habits are affected by various transitions and life circumstances.

2	**1**	**0**
Never or Almost Never	Sometimes	Always or Almost Always

After adding all the numbers you have circled, you will have a score that ranges from a low of 0 to a high of 24. Here is what those scores mean:

IF YOUR SCORE WAS FROM 0 TO 7: You are struggling to find constructive ways to use the long-term nature of your relationship to gain control over your daily health habits. Seeing the openings for this principle does take practice and patience. Make sure the messages that you are exchanging are unambiguously positive, and only then take steps to hear and appreciate the direct but ultimately caring messages that will help you curb your appetite and get you moving more.

IF YOUR SCORE WAS FROM 8 TO 16: You recognize the basics of how your relationship can operate like a fulcrum to transform the "tough love" message into better decisions about eating right and moving more. Find ways to build on this solid foundation by reinforcing the specific instances when this message encourages you to strive for more challenging goals.

IF YOUR SCORE WAS FROM 17 TO 24: You take an active approach in supporting each other to make and sustain sacrifices for your health—perhaps even to the point where they do not even seem like sacrifices anymore. Your goal is to enjoy the success you have achieved while teaming up to anticipate new challenges.

KEY POINTS FROM CHAPTER 3

- The people who make up great basketball teams, jazz trios, and theatrical troupes all manage to produce results that are far greater than the sum of their individual contributions—provided they are working from the same playbook, sheet music, or script. Our relationships are no different. Two partners can multiply their individual efforts to eat right and move more, provided they collaborate in the help they each provide and request.

- Effective collaboration in the pursuit of better health does not require boundless empathy, extensive negotiation, or a vast set of communication skills. Instead, effective support comes from translating the three bases of power that underlie all close relationships into three specific types of actions that combine to make it easier for us to be healthy than it is to be unhealthy.

- First, by knowing the Principle of Mutual Influence, partners find positive and subtle ways to strengthen each other's esteem and resolve, take initiative in modeling healthy behaviors, and monitor and capitalize on even small steps in the right direction.

- Second, by knowing the Principle of Mutual Understanding, partners recognize the value of describing the type of help they need, conveying appreciation for each other's readiness to make specific changes in their diet and exercise habits, and exchanging support that is well tailored to their individual goals.

- Third, by knowing the Principle of Long-Term Commitment, partners learn to speak candidly but compassionately about the importance of maintaining good health over the long term, draw upon their shared affection and dedication to bolster their ability to sacrifice short-term temptations for long-term gains, and discover ways to anticipate and adapt to changes in their lives that might compromise their health.

- Effective pursuit of better health is optimized when partners find ways to act on all three of these principles in their daily lives.

PART II

TEAMING UP
TO EAT RIGHT

IF YOU EAT TOGETHER,
YOU CANNOT DIET ALONE

For many people striving for a healthier weight, eating right is an essential part of their strategy. Gaining control over the calories we consume is a great idea, of course, but often the greater challenge is converting smart initial changes into a lifetime of healthy eating habits. As we demonstrated in Part I, our relationships hold the key to meeting this challenge. In the three chapters that make up Part II, we explain how the Principles of Mutual Influence, Mutual Understanding, and Long-Term Commitment enable partners to join forces in the most effective ways possible in their quest for a healthier diet. We begin with a fact that is obvious but still overlooked in most books about healthy eating: because each person in a couple is such a central part of the partner's eating environment, one person deciding to eat healthier *cannot help* but affect the other person. And the inverse is also true: deciding *not* to eat healthier *also* inevitably affects the other person. We explain how you and your partner can use this *mutual influence* to your advantage, before turning to outline how you can deepen *mutual understanding* of each other's needs for effective support in eating right, and how you can use your *long-term commitment* to make healthy food choices today that will leave you feeling healthier well into the distant future.

4

Eating Right and Mutual Influence

RECOGNIZING OUR POWER OVER WHAT OUR PARTNER EATS

"I PICTURE MYSELF BECOMING MY MOTHER." For Cathy, this was a disturbing thought. Most of her life, she had been physically fit. In high school and college, she was a member of the gymnastics team, practicing for hours each day and watching what she ate. Her mother had always been the opposite: extremely overweight, diabetic, struggling with joint trouble and breathing problems that limited her mobility. So when Cathy started noticing her own weight gain, she couldn't help but think of the future. She told her husband, Joe: "*It's scary for me because I do not want to have her health issues, even though I'm a billion miles away from those issues right now.*"

When Cathy and Joe visited our research rooms shortly after they got married, Cathy had no trouble identifying and expressing her concerns about her diet. She and Joe had been getting ready to move into a new house, and in packing up some old photographs, Cathy—now twenty-seven years old—found that she did not like comparing the person she saw in those photos with the person she saw in the mirror.

Cathy: I look at myself back then and I look at myself now—I'm not talking like high school, I'm talking about even when I first came to college. I was buff!

Joe: You were thin.

Cathy: It bothers me because there's been so much progression in what I think is a short amount of time. I have fallen into such a rut. Before, and this sounds stupid, but I would not touch fried foods. No french fries. Pizza occasionally. McDonald's? I went over a year without having one thing from McDonald's. I did not have bacon. I did not have eggs. Well, I rarely had eggs. I mean, I was so conscious and so mindful of what I was eating. Now? If it's food and it's not old or moldy or disgusting and I'm hungry? It's more "eat when you can" instead of planning meals, and it's a lot of eating out.

Cathy, like many of us, wants to eat healthier. And she knows what a nutritious diet would look like; she used to have one. But in her current life, eating right seems so hard. A social worker with a full caseload, she gets home from work late, ravenous but too tired to imagine cooking and cleaning up afterward. So it's takeout again, even though she knows that restaurant food tends to be much higher in fat and sodium than the foods she might prepare at home.

Cathy had been trying to work on this for a while, with little to show for it. It was painfully ironic that a recent experience in a class on stress management only made her feel more anxious about her increasing weight.

Cathy: It's really tough for me. When I was in the stress-management class, they were asking whether or not I accomplished my goal, which was losing ten pounds. And I hadn't lost it; I gained it. And they asked: What did you learn about this goal? And I said that setting this goal and not being able to accomplish it has made me understand that there should be nothing more important to focus on than my health. Ultimately, my eating is going to lead to health issues down the road—you know, leg problems or diabetes or whatever—because I have such crappy eating habits. And that's very bothersome to me. Because I think of me turning into my mom, and that scares me.

In terms of the stages of change that we discussed in chapter 3, Cathy is pretty far along. She absolutely knows that she has a problem, and she is committed to making a change. But, so far, actual change has proven difficult.

Joe, for his part, was sympathetic. A twenty-nine-year-old graduate student trying, and mostly failing, to finish his dissertation, Joe was not concerned about his own eating habits. With more flexible hours than Cathy, he had more time to prepare his own food, and besides, he did not have Cathy's fondness for creamy desserts. He understood his wife's concerns about her eating and her weight, though, and he wanted to do what he could to help. But they had been down this conversational path many, many times before, and his willingness to review Cathy's issues again was wearing thin. *"The problem I have,"* Joe told Cathy, *"is that we talk about it but nothing really gets done."*

As Cathy shared her fears and frustrations about her diet, Joe listened, attentive but mostly silent. As the minutes passed, however, his impatience began to leak through. He fidgeted. He sighed. When he finally broke in to speak, he started out as if he were going to offer her a solution, although she had not asked him for one. Before he could even complete that thought, however, Joe's real concern emerged. He had concluded that Cathy brings up her issues about eating so that he will take over and solve the problem for her. Joe was not eager to adopt this role.

Joe: The only thing I can suggest . . . I mean, I can't be your
willpower for you. Sometimes you ask me to try to do that, and
I don't feel comfortable because then I feel like the guy on Jenny

Jones who says, "My wife can't eat this, my wife can't eat that."
Seriously, that's how I feel when you say, "Don't let me eat dessert
tonight!" and five minutes later you say, "Let's go get ice cream."
That makes me play the bad guy, and I can't do that.

Joe is caught in a familiar bind. On the one hand, he cares about
his wife and wants to be a supportive husband. He hears Cathy wanting
to eat better, and he sincerely wants to see her meet her goals. On the
other hand, none of the ways he can think of to help seem very appealing or effective. He does not want to serve as Cathy's conscience, and
he does not want to have to be the "bad guy," taking away her treats and
the unhealthy foods she enjoys.

After eliminating those options, Joe was out of cards and feeling
frustrated. Cathy could sense it. Someone, it seemed to Joe, must be to
blame for how helpless they both felt, and he was pretty sure it wasn't
him. What he really wanted to say is *"If you want to eat healthier, then just
eat healthier, and leave me out of it!"* Instead he took a more subtle approach to saying the same thing.

Joe: The only thing I can suggest is, I can try to give up some of
those things too. I'll try. But I don't eat the sweets. I never—again,
I'm changing the subject on you—*I'm* not the one who wants to
get food late at night. I'll agree with it if you want to, but . . .

Cathy: I know and I'm not blaming you. I'm not saying that you're
at fault. I'm saying it's me. I turn into this—I'm telling you—like
totally different person.

Joe: I just don't know what I can do to help. I really don't.

Cathy: I'm not sure that there really is anything.

Compared with many couples who struggle with diet and eating
right, Joe and Cathy have so much going for them. They don't need to
be educated about the elements of a healthy diet; they already *know* what
they should be eating. They care about each other and genuinely support

each other's well-being. Moreover, they are both making important, indisputable points. Cathy, like a lot of working people, really is limited in the time that she can spend on buying and preparing healthy food. And it is reasonable for Joe to want Cathy to accept responsibility for what she eats and not expect him to be the disciplinarian. Yet somehow, despite accurate knowledge and the best intentions, they end up stuck. The sticking points of this conversation—and of countless others that they have had on this same topic—will keep Cathy from overcoming her biggest internal and external pressures when it comes to eating right.

Many couples are like Cathy and Joe, worried about their weight, knowing that they are not meeting their standards for a healthy diet, and becoming increasingly fed up with conversations that leave them feeling trapped and alone. They have a vague sense that they should be involved in each other's attempts to eat better, but are not sure where to begin, and see pitfalls at every turn. How can they get unstuck?

The first step is to apply the Principle of Mutual Influence we learned about in Part I. In this chapter you will learn to apply the Principle of Mutual Influence to your own conversations about diet and food consumption, so that you and your partner can move closer to your goals for healthy eating. As you learn how to put this principle into practice, you will be able to recognize three big traps that can make it difficult for couples to approach eating right as a team:

1. Some partners adopt the role of the *Disengager*, denying their influence on their partner and thereby missing easy opportunities to help.

2. Other partners insist on too much influence. The one trying to lose weight becomes the *Demander* or the one trying to help takes on the mantle of the *Taskmaster*—hoarding responsibility instead of sharing it.

3. Still other partners, recognizing the pitfalls of these two extremes, get stuck in the *All-or-Nothing Paradox*, paralyzed by the mistaken

idea that their only options are to take control of their partners or to withdraw.

As we examine some couples who have fallen into each of these traps, we will see that the Principle of Mutual Influence not only helps us to recognize them, but also suggests ways of avoiding or escaping them.

NOT ENOUGH INFLUENCE: THE DISENGAGER

When partners are talking together about dieting, they're not necessarily talking about dieting *together*. Faced with a spouse who wants a better diet, some people respond as if they have received an unwanted telemarketing call during dinner: *Yes, I agree with your cause, but why are you telling me about it now?* They support their partners' goals, but see no reason why they should lift a finger to help, much less join in. After all, they are not the ones who are concerned about what they eat. These are the telltale signs of the Disengager, one of the most common roles we see partners fall into when couples discuss one partner's wish to make a positive change in his or her eating behaviors.

Disengagers speak often of self-reliance. Yes, they want their partners to lose weight, but they also think that the success or failure of dieting is completely up to their partners. Some Disengagers already eat well, so they see no need to take on the burden of their partner's struggles. Other Disengagers are happy to continue with their Big Gulps and cheeseburgers, and may even feel hounded by their partner's desire to eat better. In both cases, Disengagers assume that their own behaviors and choices are irrelevant in any discussion of their partner's eating. One of our lab participants captured this point of view perfectly when, genuinely puzzled, he asked his spouse, "*How does my eating a pizza affect your diet?*"

The wife in another couple was similarly insensitive to her effects

He genuinely felt her pain, or at least tried to. He had researched her problem online and read numerous books, trying to figure out how to offer help in a way that she would accept. Her reaction was not what he hoped it would be:

W: I don't need your help. I mean, I can do it without your help.

H: That's what all the stuff says, that I'm supposed to let you deal with it on your own.

W: [talking over him] Well, the stuff's wrong. All the stuff's wrong, because you're talking to someone with the problem.

H: Well, what do you want me to do?

W: I don't know, but it doesn't have anything to do with you.

The wife told her husband that her eating problems have nothing to do with him. This is plainly false. He may not be the cause of the problems, but he is affected by her suffering, as any loving partner would be and as the Principle of Mutual Influence tells us is inevitable in a close relationship. He was willing to do whatever he could to give her what she needs, but she was having none of it, insisting that her problems were her own to solve. That's another opportunity lost. Imagine how this conversation might have been different if the wife had been able to appreciate the effects she has on her husband and the effects he might have on her. Rather than rejecting his help, she might have guided him toward things he could do that she might actually find useful.

The Principle of Mutual Influence reminds us that for couples who share their lives and their meals, remaining disengaged is not an option. Partners *are* engaged, like it or not. The choice couples face is whether to undermine each other's efforts or support them.

If Your Partner Is a Disengager

If your partner is a Disengager, you have a number of options for helping him or her make the right choice.

on her husband's eating. She was fit and she knew it; he wa trying—unsuccessfully—to shed several inches around his midsection. Her advice to him was reasonable: Eat less! But she make it easier with suggestions like this: "*You just have to control put in your mouth. Like if I go to the Cold Stone Creamery, that does that you have to get a big fat whopping cone. You can taste mine.*"

Eating right is challenging enough without having our loved throw temptation in our faces. But by denying the way their own ing can influence their partners, Disengagers are simply trying to responsibility. Their partners may have to struggle with changing habits, give up foods they love, and feel frustration and anguish, but Disengagers will not.

Think of the lost opportunities! Our partners are in the best po sible position to help us overcome obstacles and avoid temptations, help us control our eating when it might be hard to do so alone.

Imagine if the pizza-eating husband had said to his wife, "*You know what? We both could stand to lose a few pounds. How about if we just skip the pizzas at home for a while and see how we feel?*" By recognizing that his pizza absolutely does affect her ability to eat right, he might have considered a suggestion that could improve her health as well as his. Or maybe the wife who loves ice cream sees no need to cut down herself, but she might still support her husband by getting her cone when he isn't around. She might have said, "*I know that my eating ice cream reminds you of how much you love ice cream, too, so for the next six weeks, I am going to reserve my ice cream for when I go out with the girls. You and I can find another way to spend our date nights!*"

A Disengager does not have to be the partner who is in the position of providing help. Sometimes the Disengager is the person who *needs* the help. One of the saddest circumstances we see in our research is the Disengager who desperately requires support but is afraid or unwilling to ask for it. For example, one wife who visited our research rooms had been battling unhealthy eating habits, a fact she acknowledged in our labs only after some prodding by her husband.

EXPLAIN HOW YOUR PARTNER'S ACTIONS — AND INACTIONS — AFFECT YOU. If the Principle of Mutual Influence were obvious, we would not be writing this book. Sometimes our partners are simply not aware of how deeply their choices and actions affect us. In these cases, it is our responsibility to let them know, and to do it in a loving, nonjudgmental way. Avoid accusations ("You're *the one who makes it so hard for me to keep to my diet!*"). Instead, think about making a disclosure. By letting your partner know how he or she is affecting you, you are revealing something of yourself, and that can be a gift if expressed the right way.

The following example shows how a wife, frustrated by her husband's reluctance to change his own unhealthy eating habits, might handle the situation:

W: I get that you're happy with the way you eat. Really, I get it, and I'm not asking you to change. But I'm trying to change what *I* eat, and you know how hard it has been for me and how long I have been working on this. I'm literally resisting temptation *all the time,* and by the end of the day, I'm exhausted from it. So when there's fried chicken on the table, or you're sitting next to me on the couch with a brownie—sure, it's up to me to control what I eat, but those things make it so much harder. I know you don't want to make this more difficult for me than you know it already is, so let's think of ways that we can work together to make our home a place where it's easier to make healthy choices together.

H: Well, what if I only got fried chicken on the nights that you go out with your sister? Or, what if I hid the brownies somewhere where you can't find them?

Sometimes it really is that easy. By focusing on her own experience, this wife sidesteps any arguing over whether or not partners have a role to play in each other's eating. A disclosure simply states that one partner is affected by the other. Faced with a statement, rather than a criticism, the other partner has no reason to get defensive, so he or she can start volunteering to help out without losing an argument or giving in.

EXTEND AN INVITATION. Demanding involvement is not the way to go. When we make demands, our partners naturally feel constrained and start looking for a way out. Skip the demands, and extend an invitation instead. An invitation—because it leaves the decision to accept the invitation in your partner's hands—treats your partner as an equal. Even if your partner doesn't do exactly what you have invited him or her to do, many times an invitation will open up a discussion of other productive ways to join together. Try these examples for a sense of how inviting you can be:

"To get more veggies into our diet, I was thinking of hitting that farmers' market this weekend. Want to come?"

"I just got a great cookbook. Would you want to page through it together? I've already seen some low-fat dishes that we might both be interested in trying."

"Oh, this is the best salad I've ever had! Want a bite?"

The goal of extending invitations is not to manipulate your partner into performing any particular action. Rather, an invitation reinforces the message that eating healthy is something you can do together, and that might be fun to do together. With that tone in mind, your partner may be inspired to join in with suggestions of his or her own.

If You Are the Disengager

If you recognize that *you* have been a Disengager, now is the time to get involved! Once you understand the Principle of Mutual Influence, you can see that *being a team* is the best way to help your partner make the lasting changes that your partner wants to make. Teamwork does not have to look the same for every couple. For example, one husband who got it right understood that if his wife was going to change her diet, he would have to change what he ate too. In their case, this meant joining her in a program that delivered premade frozen meals to their home.

W: I like to eat stuff I'm not supposed to eat.

H: I know you like to eat stuff you're not supposed to eat. But my concern is for you and if the way these people want to help is to encourage you to eat frozen food, then that's what I want to eat.

W: Yeah, but it doesn't make me happy.

H: I understand that—

W: But I don't want to be unhappy.

H: I'm supposed to make you happy!

This husband is *engaged*. He sees that he has a role to play in his wife's progress toward a healthier weight. By joining her program—even though he may not need or want to—he has the ability to make these frozen meals, which she clearly does not like, something fun. More to the point, he is positioning himself to say that their collaboration is essential to a lifetime of good eating, and he is ready to do his part.

For the wife in a different couple, teamwork meant agreeing to what foods entered the house: "*I think when we plan our food and go grocery shopping, it's helpful to go together, because then we're making joint decisions and no one is making decisions for the other person.*"

Notice all the good things that she does in a single sentence: she treats decisions about food as something they do as a couple, she uses the word *we,* and she lets her partner know that both of them have equal responsibility for their food choices. All of this shows an appreciation for mutual influence.

If you have been the kind of Disengager who turns away help, the Principle of Mutual Influence has implications for you too. In your partner, you have a potential ally in your efforts to eat better. If you have a partner who is willing to get involved, that is a big step in the right direction and not something to be taken for granted. Does your partner know exactly what you would find most helpful? Maybe not, but your partner will never find out what you need if you don't allow anyone else to know what you are going through. And you will never find out how helpful your partner can be.

ACCEPT WHAT YOU ARE OFFERED. You may be pleasantly surprised by how much lighter a burden can be when it rests on two sets of shoulders. Consider the following couple from one of our studies, involving a husband who at long last has managed to start eating one serving of vegetables a day. *"I could eat better,"* he acknowledges reluctantly, to which his wife responds, *"Jackson, meet vegetables. Vegetables, meet Jackson. Okay, then. We've made the formal introduction now!"* She is teasing him, but in a gentle way, and he later teases her back about her tendency to prod him.

> **H:** Here's one thing I wonder: Am I eating better because I want to feel better, or do I just want to get you off my back about eating vegetables?
>
> **W:** *[laughing]* I like cooking for you and, you know, taking care of you.
>
> **H:** I know; that's why I married you.
>
> **W:** Because of my cooking?
>
> **H:** *[smiling]* Because you want to take care of me. And I'm such a screwup that I need to be taken care of!

This conversation could easily have gone differently. The husband could have demanded that his wife back off, stop with the nagging, and figure out that he just does not like vegetables. Instead, he accepts the suggestion to eat better and responds to the love that inspires his wife to want to get involved in his diet. This is an intimate moment, and it is telling that his humor in the last statement is self-deprecating rather than mean-spirited. He is grateful for the care that she offers, and she, having been reinforced by his response, is more likely to offer more of it in the future. This husband may take a while to get up to two vegetables a day, but their approach inspires confidence that he will get there eventually with her involvement.

TOO MUCH INFLUENCE: THE TASKMASTER AND THE DEMANDER

Whereas Disengagers deny that the way they eat affects their partners, those who fail to appreciate the Principle of Mutual Influence can also go to the other extreme. Rather than deny their influence, some partners insist that one partner can single-handedly make the other change the way he or she eats. These partners are engaged all right, but they have trouble with the "mutual" part of the Principle of Mutual Influence. In our research, we see this sort of misunderstanding come in two flavors.

The Taskmaster

The first flavor is the *Taskmaster.* Faced with a partner who is struggling to eat better, the Taskmaster says, "No problem! It's my job to whip you into shape!" And whipping just about covers all that the Taskmaster is willing to do. Like the Disengager, the Taskmaster is not interested in working as a team. Instead, the Taskmaster is more comfortable acting as a coach or a drill sergeant, like the wife in our studies who said the following to her unhappy husband, "*You gotta be stern. You gotta do it, baby. Do it, do it, do it! You gotta motivate yourself: 'I need to lose weight, I need to lose weight.' You can lose weight if you want to.* [pause] *Do you have anything else you want to talk about?*"

Once this wife has issued her commands, she has little else to say and is ready to move on to talking about something else. Like all Taskmasters, she hopes to induce her husband to change, but her tool kit for affecting change pretty much begins and ends with a sneaker commercial: "Just do it!" For partners who have been trying their best to "just do it" and have been frustrated by failure, this is not very useful or supportive advice.

IF YOUR PARTNER IS A TASKMASTER: The way to escape the Taskmaster trap is to take advantage of the fact that your partner really is invested in helping you eat better. That investment is a lever that you can push, gently, by recognizing the Taskmaster's good intentions and redirecting that positive energy toward behaviors that might actually be helpful.

The husband of the Taskmaster described above, for example, might have helped both of them out if he had kindly but firmly rejected her offer to change the subject. For example, when she asked if he had anything else he wanted to talk about, he might have said:

> Actually, I want to keep talking about my diet some more. The truth
> is that I already know that I need to lose weight; my motivation is
> not the problem. My problem is that I have a hard time resisting
> foods that I know I shouldn't eat. I know you want to help me eat
> better, which is great because I could really use your help.

Notice that it is possible to ask for a different sort of help without saying that the help the wife just offered is useless—even though it is. By wrapping his request in a disclosure ("*I have a problem, and here's what it is.*"), he engages with her desire to see him get healthier without criticizing what she was doing before. That's a consistent message that partners can respond to without defensiveness. In other words, the best response to the Taskmaster is an invitation to join in the task, to highlight the "mutual" in the Principle of Mutual Influence.

The Demander

The second flavor of partner who misses that mutuality is the *Demander*. Whereas the Taskmaster says to the partner trying to lose weight, "You can do it, so just do it!" the Demander *is* the person trying to lose weight, who flips this around and says, "No, *you* do it *for* me!" Demanders, recognizing how hard it is to eat right, throw up their hands and ask their partners to take the reins. Again, this request recognizes how powerfully partners affect each other, but it misses the part where this influence is mutual and shared. Instead, Demanders ask for help as a way of giving up on themselves and relinquishing control entirely. Take this wife, for example:

> I really do need to start eating healthy, and stop eating SpaghettiOs
> and ravioli and cookies and my Flying Saucers, which I haven't had
> in such a long time! Stuff like that. I do need to eat healthy. So, in
> other words, I need you to help me eat healthy.

It's telling that this wife leaps directly from stating her goal to demanding help. She skips right past her own control over what she eats, and later in the conversation she reveals why. It turns out that, while she continues to demand that her husband solve her problem, she does not actually want the help he is likely to provide.

H: I am more than willing to help you lose weight, if that is what you
   want. But like I told you before—
W: I don't want you to say, Dana, don't eat that!
H: No, I won't. But if I see you are eating something that you should
   be cutting down on, I'm going to say something.
W: But in a nice way. Don't be rude about it, because then you know
   you'll end up ticking me off and I'll end up eating it anyway.
H: That's fine. So, no more Cinnabon three times a week.
W: No, no, no! I didn't say "never." I said "cut down"!

This wife wants her husband to fix her problem, but she does not want to be part of the process herself, and she resents or rejects any of his suggestions that require sacrifices or changes on her part. So, like

Taskmasters, Demanders simply want their partners to make the problem go away, and this is rarely possible.

IF YOUR PARTNER IS A DEMANDER: Of course we want to fix our partner's problems, especially if they are standing in front of us shouting "Fix my problems!" The Principle of Mutual Influence helps us to remember that, as much as we might wish to, swooping in and changing our partner's eating habits is not in the cards. Instead, a sensitive partner will redirect the Demander's eagerness for change toward concrete behaviors that are actually doable.

Making this switch does not require a critique (*"You are just trying to make me responsible for your weight!"*) or a rejection (*"This is your problem, so leave me out of it."*). It can be as simple as asking a question. That's the approach of one husband whose wife raised the issue of her diet hoping he would fix it. He clearly wanted to, but take a look at how he goes about it:

> **H:** So what are you going to do? Because I know you have a hard time with that sort of thing. You'll go good for a few months and stop.
> **W:** What happens to me is, I'll get on a good track and then something will change. Then I won't be able to carry it over. I didn't exactly grow up in a household where anything was very disciplined, so it's hard for me to do that, you know?

This husband could have taken control as a Taskmaster and said, "Okay, so here's what you have to do . . ." Instead, he puts the control back in her hands and asks, *"So what are you going to do?"* The result is that she opens up instead of closing down, acknowledging that her family background left her poorly equipped to stick to a rigid diet plan. Later in the same conversation, he again uses questions to direct her toward making a real change:

H: So what are some of the things you'd like to add and take away
   from your diet? I mean, if we could talk about some of the things
   that you want badly . . .

W: Well, vitamins and minerals.

H: Any sort of foods? Like more nuts?

W: I would say taking out some of the alcohol would be good, and
   cakes and candies . . . And breads, I love to eat breads.

This husband has not made one suggestion or recommendation to
his wife, not a single comment that might imply that he has the power
to fix her eating. But he is still engaged, not only asking questions but
also following up with more specific questions, and she responds to that.
Asking good questions turns out to be a key to Mutual Influence, and
the best part is that it does not require that either partner be an expert
in diet, or know anything about nutrition. Asking good questions is
something that any attentive, caring partner can do. By the end of their
conversation, this wife has generated all of the answers herself, but that's
not how she sees it.

W: I don't know what to say, I want to eat better and we've outlined
   some good ways to do that!

She says that "we" have outlined good ways to eat better, and in an
important way, she's right. It took both of them—one sensitive partner
and one partner ready for change—to get to a place where progress
seems possible.

Navigating between the Taskmaster on the one hand and the Demander on the other requires that both partners give up the idea that one
or the other can fix this problem alone. Because eating is a shared activity,
changing the way either person eats has to be a shared activity as well.

THE ALL-OR-NOTHING FALLACY

We see a lot of caring partners get trapped in the space between no influence and too much influence. There's the wife whose husband wants her to monitor what he eats. She knows she could do it, but worries about the consequences.

> **W:** Well, instead of me saying, "Don't eat that" like you want me to, I'll just turn to you and be like, "Count to five before you order that and see if you still want it." I can do that for you when I'm with you. I can't be like, "Oh don't eat that," because I feel like a controlling bitch. I don't want to be that.
>
> **H:** Well, I'd rather you be a controlling bitch than me weigh two hundred and fifty pounds.
>
> **W:** Yeah, but I don't want to. I mean, that's the main problem. You're always like, "You shouldn't have let me eat that!" and I'm like, "You seem to be enjoying it." But I can't be your mom, you know?

One husband, responding to his wife's request that he help her resist the sweets she loves after dinner, makes the same point more simply: *"I'm willing to help you. But I'm not willing to deprive you either."*

These partners want to help, but they don't want to take over. They know they need to be involved in their partners' efforts to change their eating, but they imagine—correctly—that nagging and pestering their partners is unlikely to benefit the relationship. In other words, these partners have a rich and accurate sense of what NOT to do to influence their mates' eating behaviors. Unfortunately, their admirable desire to avoid common pitfalls leaves them paralyzed.

The paralysis comes from what we call the All-or-Nothing Fallacy. Like the Disengager, the Taskmaster, and the Demander, the All-or-Nothing Fallacy is a trap that arises from a misunderstanding of the

Principle of Mutual Influence. The fallacy is the idea that if we do not want to control, nag, or hector our partners into changing, then there is nothing else we can do for them. In other words, when it comes to influence, our only options are browbeating or backing off completely. It's a common belief, and many of the partners we see in our research express it directly. But it is still a fallacy, and a counterproductive one at that. Fortunately, our first principle can show you how to get beyond it.

Resolving the All-or-Nothing Paradox to Help Your Partner Eat Right

Nagging and controlling what our partners eat only seem like leading options when we forget that *we affect our partners' eating habits whether we try to control them or not.* Recognizing the Principle of Mutual Influence shines a bright light on the countless ways we can make it easier for our partners to make healthy food choices without parenting them or becoming their parole officers. The ways literally are countless, but here are a few general strategies to get you started:

SET UP THE ENVIRONMENT. Food-wise, people tend to fare poorly in settings that make bad choices easier than healthy ones. We can take this insight and turn it around on behalf of our partners; we can create environments that make *healthy* choices easier. Look around your kitchen and pantry and ask yourself how easy it is to find the unhealthy foods compared with the healthy ones:

- Is there a bowl of M&M's on the counter? Move it to the closet and replace it with a bowl of tangerines. You're not throwing out the sweets, just making them less easy to grab.
- Going shopping for your household? Think of filling your cart with fresh fruits and whole grains. If your partner wants sweets and salty snacks, he or she can still go out and get them, but you don't have to facilitate unhealthy behaviors.

- Consider the powerful fact that we all tend to finish whatever is put on our plates. Rather than heaping your partner's plate full of food, with another bowl on the table for seconds, try putting less on your partner's plate to start with, and leave the leftovers in the fridge.

If you can create a home in which healthy choices are just easier to make, your partner will find it easier to make healthy choices. And— bonus!—you'll find it easier, too.

MODEL HEALTHY BEHAVIORS. Part of setting up a healthy environment for our partners is recognizing that *we* are the most influential part of our partners' environments. The better care we take of ourselves, the better it will be for our partners' health. You may not be the one trying to lose weight, but would you be willing to cut down on desserts for a while if it would help your partner to lose weight? Your meat-and-potatoes partner might not be a fan of fresh vegetables, but those veggies might look a lot more appealing if you seem to be enjoying them. And the best way to help your partner eat smaller portions is to serve smaller portions to yourself as well. Yes, all these ways of supporting our partners require that we make sacrifices. Making sacrifices for our partner is a great way to show our love for them and our support for their health goals.

GET CREATIVE. It's one thing to say, "Eat more vegetables!" but it's quite another to say, *"Hey, honey, remember how much you like beets? I found this recipe and was hoping we could make it together. Do we have any balsamic vinegar?"* Think about ways to make healthier foods more exciting and delicious. It can be done, and here is where partnering and parenting overlap in an appropriate way.

Parents of young children often wrestle with similar challenges. *How do I get those I love and care for to eat healthy foods that they may not like?* Cookbooks for parents like *Deceptively Delicious* by Jessica

Seinfeld and *The Sneaky Chef* by Missy Chase Lapine are full of . . . well, tricks for tucking healthy ingredients into foods that kids will want to eat. It turns out that the same cooking techniques apply equally well when cooking for reluctant adults. Researching and experimenting with new techniques and recipes is a way of turning a chore into an adventure, of enticing our partners to make better choices instead of demanding them.

START SMALL. Partners who are trapped in the All-or-Nothing Fallacy assume that the only way to affect their partners is through severe behaviors like nagging, throwing out all the junk food, or monitoring their partners' every bite. In fact, relationships are a context where little things really do mean a lot. So, if you care about your partner's health, start small. Don't worry about negotiating a big agreement between you and your partner; just take the initiative on your own. You can start today if you like. Eat a bit less, or a bit better. Buy less food, or buy healthier food. Try waiting a week before you buy your favorite baked goods.

When we are trapped by the All-or-Nothing Fallacy, our options for helping our partners eat healthier look narrow and unappealing. Appreciating the Principle of Mutual Influence frees us from that trap. None of the strategies we have described here require us to talk down to our partners. They require us only to care about our partners, and to back up our feelings with actions.

KEY POINTS FROM CHAPTER 4

- Partners who struggle with their mutual influence over each other's eating typically face one of three obstacles. Some partners deny their influence on each other, missing easy opportunities to help. Other partners insist on too much influence, taking responsibility instead of sharing it. Still other couples, recognizing the pitfalls of these two extremes, get stuck in the middle, paralyzed by the mistaken idea that their only options are all or nothing. The Principle of Mutual Influence suggests ways of avoiding or escaping these traps.

- If your partner denies his or her effects on your eating (the *Disengager*), your challenge is to get your partner to recognize that the two of you influence each other, like it or not. Avoid attacks or critiques, but do try disclosing your own experience of how hard it is to eat right. Avoid demands, too, and instead consider inviting your partner to join you. And if you have been the one pushing your partner away, take a chance on accepting the support your partner has to offer as a first step toward getting the support you really need.

- If your partner is a *Taskmaster*, trying to nag or manipulate you into eating better, your goal must be to redirect that positive energy toward behaviors that might actually be supportive. Appreciate the fact that your partner wants to be involved, and then be specific about the things your partner can do that you would find helpful. On the other hand, if your partner is a *Demander*—the one who wants to make a change and is insisting that you take over—then your job is to remember that you cannot solve your partner's issues alone, as much as you might like to. Try asking questions of your partner instead, helping your partner to generate solutions on his or her own.

- Some partners who want to be supportive feel trapped between two bad options: taking responsibility for policing their partners' eating, or being entirely uninvolved. This is the *All-or-Nothing Fallacy*. Appreciating the Principle of Mutual Influence reveals this to be a false choice. The many ways that partners can support each other's goals without nagging or controlling include setting up healthy food environments and modeling healthy eating behaviors. Because mutual influence between partners is so strong, small changes in the behavior of either partner cannot fail to have ripple effects, so make them positive ones!

PLANNING FOR CHANGE

Within an intimate relationship, partners have enormous influence on each other when it comes to what, when, and how much they eat. In this chapter, we have described how couples can recognize and use that influence to promote better eating habits and further each partner's diet goals. Before moving on, this final section invites you to think about the mutual influence between you and your partner right now.

Each of the statements below describes something that successful couples do to support each partner's efforts to eat right. For each one, consider how well you and your partner engage in this behavior, and how easy or difficult it will be for the two of you to make any needed improvements.

1. We appreciate how *our own actions and choices* affect the foods we both eat.

    _____ This is a real strength for us. We do not need to make changes in this area.

    _____ We could improve in this area, and we think it will be easy to do so.

    _____ We could improve in this area, but we think it will be difficult to do so.

2. We consider eating healthier to be *a shared activity* that we approach as a team.

    _____ This is a real strength for us. We do not need to make changes in this area.

    _____ We could improve in this area, and we think it will be easy to do so.

    _____ We could improve in this area, but we think it will be difficult to do so.

3. We *accept the help and support* that each has to offer.

    _____ This is a real strength for us. We do not need to make changes in this area.

    _____ We could improve in this area, and we think it will be easy to do so.

____ We could improve in this area, but we think it will be difficult to do so.

4. We have made *concrete, specific efforts* to improve our shared food environment, for example by making sure healthier foods are easily available and unhealthy foods more difficult to access inside our home.

____ This is a real strength for us. We do not need to make changes in this area.

____ We could improve in this area, and we think it will be easy to do so.

____ We could improve in this area, but we think it will be difficult to do so.

5. We have searched for *creative ways to incorporate healthier food choices* into our lives.

____ This is a real strength for us. We do not need to make changes in this area.

____ We could improve in this area, and we think it will be easy to do so.

____ We could improve in this area, but we think it will be difficult to do so.

If you found yourself marking the first answer a lot, then you and your partner clearly appreciate the Principle of Mutual Influence and have been exploiting that understanding to reinforce each other's efforts to eat right.

If your responses tend toward the second answer, then real change is in sight. Now that you understand how the Principle of Mutual Influence works, you and your partner have a number of great ways to meet your goals for a healthier diet, and there is nothing stopping you from working together to make those improvements happen.

If you found yourself often marking the third answer, then you and your partner may understand the Principle of Mutual Influence but still recognize that making that influence work for you in your own lives will not be easy. Consider reviewing this chapter again with the goal of identifying concrete steps that you can take today—and remember that even small changes can have big effects. You and your partner may also face challenges that go beyond recognizing your mutual influence. We address some of those challenges in the next chapter.

5

Eating Right and Mutual Understanding

DISCOVERING WHAT OUR PARTNERS REALLY NEED

BBY, A FORTY-TWO-YEAR-OLD EXECUTIVE ASSISTANT, has been married for twelve years to Dean, a thirty-nine-year-old freelance photographer and documentary filmmaker. All the information that we collected from Abby and Dean indicates they are quite happy in their relationship and that they communicate well—at least until she voices her concerns about being overweight. Abby has struggled with her weight and eating habits off and on for several years now and Dean, for his part, has struggled with knowing exactly how to respond. Usually, they opt to simply avoid the issue, but in our study Abby volunteered this topic as an area of personal concern and she turned to Dean for help. Here is how their conversation began:

> **Abby:** It's important to me that you support me, and I think you do that.
>
> **Dean:** How do I need to do that? Tell you that you look good? Tell you you're not fat, you know, when you say you are?

We have learned a lot already. Abby implies that our first principle—the Principle of Mutual Influence—is alive and well in their relationship. She knows that Dean affects her and how she feels, and she expresses her appreciation for his support. But even though both partners have told us that this issue is in no way a source of tension in their relationship, Dean already seems frustrated by Abby's tendency to say she is fat. Their positions rapidly become polarized, a pretty good sign that our second principle—the Principle of Mutual Understanding—has yet to make an appearance.

Abby: I just need you to be honest with me . . .

Dean: Right. Tell you you're not fat when you say you are. [Tell you to] eat the good stuff that you need to.

Abby: And just don't give me a hard time when I make self-disparaging remarks.

Dean: When you say that you're fat when you're not, that's wrong. That's not helping you.

Abby: Well, I do have a problem and sometimes I feel like that you . . . that you, in trying to make me feel better about myself, you kind of act like it's not there, and it is.

Dean: Well, it's not there for me. I know it's there for you. But you've got to admit that there isn't something wrong with you, that you're not fat. I mean there's nothing wrong with you. You're not different from . . . you're no heavier than anyone else. I mean, you want to lose weight. That's fine. I understand you're working on it. But to say "I'm ugly, I'm fat," I mean, you say a self-disparaging remark. You know it's not true. There's nothing wrong with you.

Abby: Well, there is some truth to it.

Dean: I understand about wanting to stay healthy and wanting to lose weight and all that, but to say that "I'm ugly, I'm fat" is not true. And even if you don't want to hear that from me, you need to know that is true.

Abby: Well, it's nice that you want to say that. But anyway . . .

Dean: Do you think you look good now?

Abby: No.

Dean: Wrong! Wrong answer. I mean, that actually is a question with a right and wrong answer, and that is just wrong.

Abby: Well, how? What I think isn't necessarily wrong, or at least how I feel isn't wrong.

Dean: It is wrong, because you're still attractive now.

Abby: Well, my opinion isn't wrong, okay? Opinions aren't "right" or "wrong" in that case. It's how you feel.

Dean: You need to feel better, too. Yes, that's true. But the opinion is wrong. You look good. You just do.

Abby is overweight, feels bad about it, and wants Dean to support healthy eating habits. But Dean does all he can to convince Abby that the negative portrait she draws of herself is wrong, hoping his protests will convey how attractive he finds her. Alas, this registers not as encouragement or motivation to eat better, but as invalidation of Abby's goals and perceptions of herself. Punished by Dean's praise, Abby is unlikely to want to repeat this conversation anytime soon. Why bother?

Because mutual understanding is so pivotal to the success of any couple's quest to eat right, we have studied many couples like Abby and Dean to understand why partners misread each other when they talk about changing the way they eat. We have discovered that many partners, by misusing the Principle of Mutual Understanding, fall into three main traps that hinder each other's efforts to eat better:

1. The *Charmer,* who offers plenty of reassurance but little practical support. The Charmer's fallback position—*Why change? I think you look great!*—sounds like exactly the thing many of us would love to hear, when in fact it invalidates our sincere efforts to change.

2. The *One-Trick Pony,* who works hard to offer useful support but has a very limited arsenal for doing so. The One-Trick Pony offers

up solutions that have worked for him or her in the past, but, often out of frustration, fails to adapt them to what the partner actually needs.

3. The *Waffler*, who seeks help but then rejects it. Not yet ready to make real changes in his or her eating habits, the Waffler is plenty ready to ask the partner for help but finds little of value in those suggestions, regardless of how good they might be.

"YOU LOOK GREAT": THE CHARMER

Mutual understanding, the centerpiece of our second principle, isn't the equivalent of mutual affection. This has been one of our most surprising research findings. Two people can feel really confident about their relationship and love each other unconditionally, yet still misunderstand each other—and even be completely stumped—when it comes to being advocates for each other's health. And, more surprising still, one person's expressions of affection can actually *interfere with* the partner's ability to make healthy food choices. How could this be?

Abby and Dean are a prime example of this kind of puzzling exchange. Most conversations involving Charmers are not as contentious as theirs, but all involve the attempted delivery of two contradictory messages. One message is definitely worth keeping: *I love you and I think you're incredible. Please try to see yourself as the person I adore.* The other message, however, needs closer examination: *Your opinion is wrong. What you want is not important. Your eating habits are fine. Don't change.* The Charmer's first message is so captivating that it often manages to engulf the second one, and so it is extremely important to step back and ask how an overabundance of praise can hinder good communication about health and fitness.

One woman in our study, like many people we have seen, wanted to lose weight, cut down on unhealthy snacks and desserts, and feel better about herself. She reported being in reasonably good shape, but expressed deep concern about ending up like her parents, who were both overweight and suffered from diabetes, high cholesterol, and high blood pressure.

> **W:** I'm not the skinny-minny and everything else I used to be. So hopefully if I start working out and [eating better] I might notice a difference and feel better about myself.
> **H:** I love you just the way you are, honey.
> **W:** I just don't like—
> **H:** I don't care what you look like. I love *you*.
> **W:** Yeah, but—
> **H:** Whatever makes *you* happy. Just, you know—don't do it because of *me,* do it for yourself.

Acceptance from a doting husband. What's not to like? Unfortunately, love alone is not going to get the job done here.

Two years later, we watched as the same husband handed a tissue to his crying wife, now claiming to be almost twenty pounds heavier and more concerned than ever about her health. Underscoring the tremendous influence of our social circles, she explained how her coworkers were baking delicious treats several days a week for the office and how she felt powerless to resist them. Losing weight now would allow her to recover more quickly after they have a baby, she said, and yet she saw how easy it would be to gain *another* twenty pounds over the next two years, and twenty pounds more after that—just like her mom. Her husband again emphasized how much he cared for her and how she, not her weight, was his highest priority.

> **H:** But why do you want to lose weight? *Why?*
> **W:** *[dabbing her eyes]* For myself, for you, for . . . I don't know!
> **H:** Well, if you're doing it for yourself, that's fine. But don't do it for me. I mean, if you're doing it for me, that's just silly. It's something you've gotta do for yourself. The only reason I would want you to lose weight is if you got unhealthy, all right? If you had, I don't

know, heart problems or something. I mean, you are not unhealthy. I really think you are fine the way you are.

W: But also I am not happy with *myself* right now either. I can't make excuses. I just need to do it. I don't know.

H: I don't care. I really don't care. You are *fine* the way you are. I don't care. I mean, in terms of these people bringing all this food to work? Just, I don't know, bring something yourself so, you know, when they are eating their chocolate cupcakes and everything you break out one of those rice cakes or something . . .

This woman is stuck, desperate, and confused. Good solutions have been hard to come by for more than two years now. And when she turns to her husband for the help she needs, she receives what *seems* like a lovely response: *You are fine the way you are. I love* you. But in this situation, it's not productive.

An unwitting coconspirator in this dilemma, the husband is equally baffled about what to do and what it will take for his wife to start eating right. After all, her weight is not a problem from his point of view. According to him, she is fighting a battle that does not need to be fought—a battle that exists only in her mind. And if she is so upset about it—as she clearly seems to be—why doesn't she just do something about it?

He is being the Charmer, professing his unwavering love but coming up short when it comes to delivering the emotional support and practical solutions his wife actually needs to eat right. It's a no-win situation. The Charmer's wife is unable to articulate her needs and the Charmer is unable to realize the limitations of his praise. The paradox of the Charmer is that his intentions of support actually end up having a negative effect.

Praise usually inspires us and makes us feel good, but when it contradicts what we are trying to accomplish it can drive us away from our goals. Mutual understanding is merely an illusion for these couples; real support is in short supply, with each person operating exclusively from his or her own frame of reference. Mutual *mis*understanding reigns, but the lack of support is never noticed because it comes wrapped in a dazzling package of charm and affection.

Meanwhile, the Charmer's partner, wanting to eat better, can feel invalidated and diminished, ultimately questioning the Charmer's sincerity. Negotiating these different perspectives can be unwieldy. After being told how great she looked, the wife in the following couple rejected the flattery—a sure sign of being in a trap. Notice how this wife, so troubled by her weight gain, referred to herself in the third person:

W: Let's see. We've been together, what, five years now? I think I've gained a total of twenty-eight pounds in five years. That's extremely upsetting and disturbing to somebody, that's all. So I just want to lose weight, okay? And I feel like I try, but I just get nowhere.

H: I just don't think you need to lose weight. You look good the way you are.

W: No! Because even sometimes, like, when I try stuff on and I'm like, "How do I look?" you're like, "eh" and I'm like, "I look chubby, don't I?" and you say "yeah." See, I don't want to look chubby when I try stuff on . . . I just don't feel like you're always honest with me. I think, like, you just get frustrated.

Clearly a Charmer, this husband went on to say, "See, I think you look great," and, later, "I think you look marvelous, baby," to which his wife responded, "Oh, be quiet," and "Oh, shut up." The friction is unmistakable. The problem is not that the husband is being dishonest. The real problem is that he can't fathom her point of view—and she can't figure out a productive way to transform his praise into the empathy she needs.

If Your Partner Is a Charmer
The first key to escaping this trap is for partners to recognize that their two different perspectives are in conflict. Neither perspective is

objectively right or wrong. Believing—as the Charmer does—that the partner looks great is a completely legitimate opinion. And wanting to eat better and slim down is an equally justified stance for the Charmer's partner to take. But both views being valid doesn't mean that they're both good road maps for progress. And as we saw in the first example above—"*I don't care. I really don't care. You are fine the way you are. I don't care*"—Charmers often become even more insistent in their vague praise as the partners begin to struggle.

The Principle of Mutual Understanding suggests several specific ways to work with a Charmer so that these two messages can be pulled apart:

ACCEPT THE PRAISE. A real strength of the Charmer is his or her ability to offer praise. Because this praise is too general ("*You're fine the way you are.*"), it is tempting to skip past it and redirect the focus onto your more specific concern ("*Yes,* but *I am not happy with the way I look*" or "But *I do not want to end up eating like my mother*" or "But *even you say I look chubby when I try on clothes*"). Rejecting praise misses an opportunity for connection and a chance to express appreciation for the relationship that you and your partner share. "Yes, but" comments tend to bring about defensiveness, whereas "yes, and" comments invite collaboration and opportunities for deeper understanding. This hypothetical example shows how this might go:

W: I need to stop snacking so much. There are times when I feel like it's just totally out of control for me.

H: It's not so big a deal. I think you look pretty great.

W: Well, that's nice of you to say, and obviously your opinion matters more to me than anybody else's. I want to do all I can to keep looking great, for you and for me. I want to be healthy and I really want to eat right so I can keep looking good.

H: Okay, so, *how?*

Had this wife said, "*But it is a big deal. I really need to stop snacking!*" this husband probably would have persisted in minimizing the issue ("*Seriously, you look fine*") or the difficulty of the task ("*So, just try to cut back, then*"), closing off further dialogue. But, by accepting her husband's praise, she has prevented her husband from becoming defensive. She is now ready to ask him to channel his attention toward the more important task at hand, and he is more likely to hear this now.

FOCUS ON YOUR SPECIFIC GOALS. Part of the Charmer's repertoire is to stay "on message," much like a politician running for office. In the previous example, we can easily imagine the Charmer continuing to insist he is right ("*You look fine! Don't change for me! I do not care how you look!*"). Getting to a real exchange about the issue involves choosing not to argue at the general level but instead discussing specific future plans. When affirming the praise in this message is not enough, focusing on the personal importance of the changes themselves can move the conversation forward: "*I guess the issue for me is not so much whether I am changing for you or for me. The reason is not so important as much as just the knowledge that I am eating a healthier balanced diet. I would like us to do that together.*" Or "*Okay, maybe I am not fat or overweight in your eyes, and I appreciate your saying that. We may see it differently and there's no sense arguing about it. Even still, I would like to cut back on snacks and sodas just as a matter of general principle. And if you could help with that it would make it so much easier for me.*"

DISCOVER WHAT YOU'RE DOING TO MAKE YOUR PARTNER RESISTANT AND DEFENSIVE. The strength and persistence of the Charmer's message suggest that he or she may be feeling pressured or threatened. What's going on here? Perhaps your Charmer needs reassurance about his own eating habits or appearance. Or maybe the Charmer feels that you are blaming him for your bad eating habits, or he senses that you are asking him to be in charge of getting your weight back on track. Challenged in this way, any of us might become defensive and hide behind platitudes.

Perhaps it is difficult for your partner to set aside his image of you as a young, svelte, sexy person. Or maybe your partner has heard you complain one too many times about failing to eat right, without your putting forth any real effort to make the change.

One or more of these unspoken feelings may be stirring up the resistance you are now facing. Ask gentle, probing questions to help you soften this resistance. Then, cultivate the support you need by engaging the Charmer on his or her own terms. With this in mind, we can revisit an earlier conversation:

> **H:** I understand about wanting to stay healthy and wanting to lose weight and all that, but to say that "I'm ugly, I'm fat" is just not true. And even if you don't want to hear that from me, you need to know that's true.
>
> **W:** Well, it's nice that you want to say that—really nice—and that really helps me to feel good about myself and good about us. So, do all those self-disparaging remarks I make just drive you nuts?
>
> **H:** Well, yeah, because they're not true, and you always say those things when you're feeling really bad about yourself. It already bothers me to see you that way, and then when you *criticize* yourself, that just makes it even worse. And, I gotta say, you're kinda dragging *me* down in the process.
>
> **W:** I guess I say those things so I can let you know how *bad* I'm feeling about myself. But if I focus more on just wanting to be healthy and less on just putting myself down, do you think you could keep encouraging me to do the right things, and eat the right things?

The details of any one conversation are less important than the general point: The Charmer may be digging in his heels, but not without good reason. Understanding that reason, and how you might be contributing to it, are important steps toward breaking through the Charmer's pretense of support.

If You Are the Charmer

If, on the other hand, *you* tend to be a Charmer when your partner talks about improving his or her eating habits, you may be creating a trap that makes it harder for your partner to be healthier and happier. Here are some things you can do to avoid this trap:

RECOGNIZE THAT YOUR PARTNER IS STRUGGLING WITH PARTS OF HIM- OR HER-SELF THAT ARE UNPLEASANT. Most of us embrace the familiar or comfortable parts of our partner's personality. But for support to be valuable we have to appreciate who our partner is *and* who they are trying to become. One husband we watched was very good at fusing these two parts of his wife's identity. At first he sounds like a Charmer, but when push comes to shove, he knows that what his wife needs is an ally.

> Look, the first thing I want you to know is that I think you're perfect, okay? And that I am happy with you in every possible way. You're beautiful, you're wonderful, and I know I'm just lucky to be with you. So let me just put that out there, okay? But if you're telling me you're not happy with how you look and the way we're eating, then, you know, that is a problem. And we need to solve that problem.

WORK ON UNDERSTANDING THE PROBLEM, NOT FIXING IT. If you are like most Charmers, you feel "put on the spot," and pressured to magically improve your partner's eating habits. "You look marvelous just the way you are!" is an easy response and, as default strategies go, it's a pretty good one. But when your partner is questioning his or her appearance or way of eating, you're better off finding a new tactic. Your usual expressions of affection turn out to be a weak substitute for the more specific sort of understanding that your partner needs. Fortunately, fostering understanding in relationships doesn't require some ingenious brand of empathy—just simple thoughtful responses.

Recall our earlier example in which the wife said, "*I think I've gained a total of twenty-eight pounds in five years. That's extremely upsetting and disturbing to somebody, that's all. So I just want to lose weight, okay? And I feel like I try, but I just get nowhere.*" Feeling pressured to deal with all this angst and frustration, her husband played the charm card: "*I just don't think you need to lose weight. You look good the way you are.*" When your partner expresses strong negative emotions about his or her weight or eating habits, you, too, can feel upset, and therefore feel pressured to put a patch on the problem. Now neither of you is functioning at your best, and progress will stall. Better to maintain some degree of neutrality, as a concerned friend might, by being engaged while still remaining reasonably objective. Try a more neutral response, like, "*Okay, take me through it. Tell me what you think is going on.*" This avoids the obvious hurdle, positioning yourself to be helpful. As the partner of someone struggling to be healthier, you do not need to have all the answers or all the solutions—but you are perfectly positioned to guide your partner to a better understanding of that struggle.

"BUT IT WORKED FOR ME!": THE ONE-TRICK PONY

Couples striving to eat right often get stuck in a loop, with partners professing real commitment to healthier eating but relying too heavily on their own perspectives. For example, we watched as one wife repeatedly championed tomatoes as the solution to her husband's finally getting his eating habits under control, to which he replied, "*Tomatoes are just not the be-all and end-all of vegetables, Katie!*" She replied, "*No, but I eat a lot of them,*" before lobbying on behalf of her other favorites: green beans, cauliflower, and carrots.

At one point the husband said, with obvious sarcasm, "*No, no, no. It's all tomatoes! I know, I know! That's all it is!*" Distracted momentarily, the wife jumped back in by suggesting, "*Um, cucumbers?*" which the husband just ignored.

This couple has fallen into another common trap. The wife, for her part, really wants to be helpful. Her husband has reached out to her, and she sees him struggling. She wants him to eat right, and she wants to help ensure this happens. She believes, correctly, that eating more vegetables is an indispensable element in a well-rounded diet. But when she offers up her one precious nugget of wisdom that she thinks will work, he rejects it. Now she is stuck: how can *she* help a person who does not want to be helped? The husband wants—and needs—his wife's help to eat right, and he genuinely appreciates her efforts. On the other hand, her wayward and self-centered suggestions leave him feeling discounted and misunderstood. So now he is stuck, too: how can *he* accept help from a person who is not being helpful? She is being the One-Trick Pony, using and reusing her one great suggestion without appreciating the possibility that he may need something different. She questions whether he is really serious about eating better, while he doubts whether she can tailor her support to his particular problem.

This couple has discovered for themselves what we have discovered in countless couples: Knowledge simply isn't enough. There is a chasm between having good ideas for eating right and actually translating them into better eating habits. The partners have not enlisted each other as allies, and they have not cultivated each other as real collaborators. Looking at a few more examples of this trap will help explain why it happens and how couples can engage the Principle of Mutual Understanding to escape it.

One wife in our study had struggled with her weight for a few years but wanted it known that "*I mean, it's not like I'm obese.*" Her husband agreed and accurately noted, "*I know. But you're not happy with your body . . .*" and then tried to encourage her to see the virtues of prepared frozen foods from a commercial weight-loss program that had worked for him in the past. He really liked the fact that these meals allowed for close monitoring of portion sizes and easy cooking in the microwave oven. She was open to this idea in principle, but was not nearly as thrilled with how the food tasted.

H: It's just really nice to know . . . "beep, beep, beep" and boom, it's
   ready to eat.

W: It just tastes so blah.

H: That's what cayenne pepper's for!

W: But then I feel very unsatisfied and I just start snacking.

H: No, listen, that's what the cayenne pepper's for! You need to get
   into the pepper aisle there to the left of the cabinet. That'll spice it
   up a bit. Hot sauce and garlic will fix anything!

He ignored her emotional reaction as he restated his proposed solution, without considering how it might be adapted to work specifically for her. This is the One-Trick Pony, trying to help but using only his own limited perspective to offer solutions. The same trap engulfs this couple below, leaving them both stuck.

W: Maybe you could just go to Weight Watchers meetings for a
   couple of weeks.

H: *[silent, uncomfortable]*

W: You don't want to.

H: That'll make me feel even *fatter.*

W: Well, that's how *I* did it—I don't know!

This wife was trying to be helpful, but by relying too much on her own experiences she inadvertently overlooked the insecurity that was affecting his choices.

At the root of this trap is the faulty assumption that, because both partners share the goal of eating well, they must pursue this goal in the same way. The One-Trick Pony assumes that she and her partner are alike when it comes to eating, but gets tripped up when putting a plan into action. The problem with this assumption, of course, is that two people in a relationship may have vastly different approaches to eating right. Here are just a few examples of those differences that we have seen:

- One person wants to make sweeping changes to the family diet; his partner thinks that simply cutting down a bit on red meat and eating more fish and vegetables will be sufficient.

- One person benefits from keeping a food log and monitoring her appetite and calories closely; the partner can easily make and follow a plan and does not see the point of such detailed record-keeping.

- One person needs a lot of help and support to eat right; her partner is willing to provide the support but prefers not to have her involved in what he eats.

- One person is committed to a healthier diet and serious weight loss; the partner, equally overweight, is willing to go along but is not nearly as concerned or motivated.

In situations like these, neither partner is really right or wrong. One person can say tomato, and the other person can say to*mah*to, without calling the whole thing off. But failing to appreciate differences like these sets the stage for a great deal of misunderstanding and miscommunication. Often, when we try to reconcile these differences, we draw from our own perspectives and experiences. Yet, as the above examples suggest, the resulting support and advice—*Just eat tomatoes! Use cayenne pepper! Try the approach that worked for me!*—end up being anything but supportive. The Principle of Mutual Understanding reminds us that we have to work *with* our partners. The "trick" that works for us may not work for our partners, and so the challenge is to set this trick aside and discover how we can bring out the best in our partners on their own terms.

If You Are a One-Trick Pony

Offering your partner reasonable advice and guidance for eating better only to have it be rejected can be frustrating. But if you find that your suggestions are ignored or dismissed, you just might be a One-Trick Pony. You need to loosen the grip on your preferred solutions and, instead, help your partner discover the strategies likely to work best *for him or her.* You may not be the sole cause of this particular problem, but there are many ways you can be the cause of the solution:

ENCOURAGE YOUR PARTNER TO EXPRESS HIS OR HER CONCERNS. Sometimes we jump in with solutions that work for us because our partner is uncomfortable opening up about his or her feelings. Respect this, and recognize that your partner might feel exposed when discussing the eating habits he or she wants to change. Listening will open up communication, while delivering strong opinions will close it down. A key part of your task is to make your partner feel comfortable and safe. Take a look at the following example:

> **W:** *[quietly]* [I need to eat better and lose weight,] but it's not really
> something I want to discuss. It's just embarrassing . . . I don't
> know. Even though you are my husband and I talk to you about
> everything, I just don't prefer to talk to you about *this.* Because it's
> so—it's . . . we've talked about it before, and there's just not much
> to talk about.
> **H:** *[nodding, also quiet]* Yeah, okay. Is this something you find yourself
> thinking about a lot?
> **W:** Yeah, actually I do . . . .

Here the husband was able to sidestep what might have felt like rejection and, by asking a question that would get his wife closer to her own feelings, helped to keep the conversation open and productive. Moments like these remind us that good support is indeed personal and intimate.

UNDERSTAND WHERE YOUR PARTNER IS STRUGGLING. Suggesting practical ways to eat better implies that there are simple, practical solutions to be had. But surely, your partner already *knows* several good solutions and is just struggling to implement them. Working to understand the struggle, and helping your partner discover ways to overcome the urges and temptations, is the better way forward:

> Sounds to me like you are already doing a lot of the right things: drinking more water, snacking on fruit and vegetables. All that is really good. But are you finding it hard to keep on track now? Like, what do you see as your rough spots?

ASK QUESTIONS THAT DEEPEN UNDERSTANDING. Devote your questions and support efforts to understanding, from your partner's frame of reference, why healthy eating is hard right now and how he or she is making sense of this puzzle. Unless your partner "owns" the solution, it's not going to become part of his or her daily routine of healthy eating.

LISTEN CLOSELY TO THE WORDS YOUR PARTNER IS CHOOSING. When your partner is trying to discover the best ways to eat right, listen closely to the words he or she uses to express that experience. Our examples above show how many such words—"discouraged," "not happy," "overwhelming," and "miserable"—were spoken but ignored. Words like these are like gifts that give you special access to your partner, and really hearing them will allow you to be more effective in providing support.

When your partner says something like, "*My weight is really upsetting me now, and I don't know what to do about it,*" this probably isn't the time to rush in with your favored solutions. Naturally we are tempted to respond to the second part of statements like this, using our own frames of reference, but the underlying emotion is really the better place to focus. Better to say something simple that acknowledges the experience as he or she has expressed it: "*Well, I'm sorry to hear you're upset. Can you help me understand what's going on?*"

ASSUME THAT YOUR PARTNER IS SMART ENOUGH AND COMPETENT ENOUGH TO MAKE PROGRESS. Offering practical solutions for eating and dieting woes may imply that your partner is unable to come up with these solutions by himself or herself. Few of us respond well to this implication, so wield solutions with extreme care. Instead, actively look for ways to put some supportive scaffolding around the efforts your partner is already putting in place.

PRAISE, DON'T JOKE. Pessimism and doubt are already burdening your partner, so disapproval from the one person who should be offering support strikes especially hard. Praise and encouragement motivate health-related changes, whereas criticism and warnings compromise our efforts to be healthier. Keep away from jokes about weight and eating habits, which are often interpreted as criticism.

> **H:** The reason this is a big deal just for me, just personally, is that
> Jeremy is over there and he's like 185 or 180 pounds or whatever,
> and he's all ripped or whatever, and *I'm* just a lazy slob.
> **W:** *[laughing]* Well, you are his *big* brother!
> **H:** Not funny.

REINFORCE PROGRESS. As you learned from our discussion of stages of change in chapter 3, deciding to eat right is not an all-or-nothing proposition, like flipping a switch. Your partner might think about it for a while, mention it to you a few times, put some healthy recipes on the refrigerator, decide not to do it because work is too stressful, and then finally take the plunge—and then waver again. Supporting your partner's healthy eating requires you to understand where he or she is in this back-and-forth process. Those repeated comments about wanting to make significant changes in eating are like the test runs that precede a leap into the deep end of a pool. Building up your partner's courage, then, is going to be a lot more effective than disparaging the aborted attempts.

If Your Partner Is a One-Trick Pony

If you're on the receiving end of ineffective support, you, too, are in the trap. The help you are receiving is not the help you need to eat right. Your unique challenge is to validate the positive elements in the support your partner is offering, while shaping it to better meet your needs.

Earlier we saw an example in which one husband skillfully walked the fine line between rejecting his wife's support and acknowledging its possible value: "*I can't put it into that framework. I mean, maybe it's possible, but I can't do it right now. I'm not in a place right now where I can think about it in that way.*" Where outright rejection of the support ("*Stop already with the positive affirmations!*") would have closed off further discussion, this approach instead invites the partner to stay involved and brainstorm better ideas. And by focusing inward on what he was feeling, rather than outward on the inadequacy of the suggestions she was offering, he increased the odds that he would be understood on his terms.

"I KNOW I NEED TO, BUT I DON'T *WANT* TO": THE WAFFLER

Knowing glances and soft voices, words ripe with shared private meaning, a consoling embrace after a rough day: communication alone determines how well relationship partners understand each other. For all its virtues, though, communication is murky and imperfect, and doubly so when couples set out to make the hard choices that will enhance their eating habits. Charmers and One-Trick Ponies each have their unique ways of ignoring or misinterpreting our intentions, but miscommunication is just as likely when the very messages that *we* send in our quest for help are ambiguous and even contradictory.

The *Waffler*, the main culprit in our third and final barrier to mutual understanding, vows to eat right and asks the partner for help, only to then turn away the very support he or she receives. Declaring the need to make major changes on the one hand, while resisting advice and encouragement on the other, the Waffler sows confusion while struggling to find the confidence he or she needs to take the first steps toward healthy eating.

Note that the Waffler introduces us to a fundamentally different kind of misunderstanding. Charmers and One-Trick Ponies have partners who are asking for help, and fumble when attempting to *provide* that help to their partners. Wafflers need help, but they create problems for *themselves,* either in the way they solicit support or in the way they respond once it is delivered.

The following couple illustrates this kind of misunderstanding. The woman reports being overweight and unhappy with her appearance, and when she states, "*I really eat awful. I'm lazy. I'm going to die at an early age if I don't quit . . . My body is—man, I'm not a healthy individual,*" it's hard to disagree. She turns to her partner for help, and is unusually fortunate in being married to a man who, having himself shed over 100 pounds on his own, works hard to help her.

H: You don't eat vegetables, so, you know, it's hard for you.

W: I hate vegetables.

H: I started eating rice cakes.

W: *[shuddering with disgust]* Ugh.

H: See, you haven't learned to diet . . . . And you need to cut down on your Pepsi, too. See, that's where a lot of your weight's coming from.

W: No, you don't understand! My Pepsi's like cigarettes to me!

H: Yeah, what you're saying is you want to do this but you're not *willing* to do it.

W: Well, I'm not giving up soda, simple as that.

H: Look, I'll help you, okay? But you are going to have to stick with it, too.

W: *[annoyed]* I will.

H: I just wish I could manage to get you to eat vegetables. I mean, they're *good!* You should give 'em a try. Like green beans and corn?

W: *[shakes head no]*

H: And spinach?

W: *[shakes head no]*

H: It's *good!* Have you even tried them lately? I mean, I hated spinach until last year.

W: No.

H: You might like my spinach quiche, though! I'm going to make it and have you try it.

W: I doubt it. I'll try it, but—

H: You don't even taste the spinach! You taste jalapeño jack cheese. And the onions.

W: Well, let's just forget it, okay? None of this is very appetizing for me.

A CDC statistic waiting to happen, this woman is unhealthy and eating poorly, and she knows she needs to make big changes soon if she is going to get her health, her weight, and her appearance back under control. She reaches out to an understanding partner. This man is not perfect—you can see where he slips into being a Taskmaster and a One-Trick Pony—but he cares about her, offers optimistic explanations for her plight (e.g., "*You haven't learned to diet*"), avoids browbeating her with his sensible firsthand knowledge about healthy eating, and offers good emotional and practical support. And yet she resists the very support she wants and needs. The problem is not with the support he provides as much as it is with how she requests and receives that support.

By asking for but dismissing help, the Waffler creates misunderstanding, essentially saying, "*I know I need to eat better, and I know I will need my partner to get mobilized. But all the help and encouragement that my partner gives me fails to recognize how hard this is, my special circumstances, how I expect to be treated, and what I am and am not willing to do to make these changes. Eat a vegetable? Stop drinking Pepsi!? What's it going to take before I get some decent support around here?!*" The Waffler adds condition after condition to the help that he or she would deem acceptable, presenting a smaller and smaller target for his or her partner to hit. And when the partner inevitably misses the target, the Waffler can only conclude, "*My partner just doesn't understand."* In reality, a more accurate conclusion should be, *"I am making it difficult for my partner to understand me."* As this pattern continues unchecked, the partner's hope and concern gradually diminish, leaving him or her to agree with the Waffler: *"You were right after all, I just don't understand."*

The Waffler contributes to misunderstanding in three ways: first, by requesting help before resolving to really change; second, by making the request in language that is unclear or loaded with emotion; and third, by resisting the partner's responses to the request. Getting some perspective on these three points strengthens mutual understanding and allows support to flow.

If You Are a Waffler

If you have a tendency to waffle like this, what can you do?

ASK FOR HELP ONLY WHEN YOU ARE READY TO MAKE GOOD USE OF IT. Know where you are in the stages of change, and accept the possibility that you are not yet ready to make lasting changes to your diet. Because you want to do this right—and you want to do it just once—you would be wise to choose the right time to advance toward a higher level of change. Take some time to sort out the issues for yourself, and consider whether you want to strengthen your resolve. By letting your partner know that you're contemplating this change—and maybe even that you're struggling a bit and not quite ready to make big changes—you are helping your partner to *understand* you. On the other hand, as with the boy who cried wolf, inviting your partner's support before you're ready to make good use of it may mean that it won't be there when you finally *are* ready to eat right.

The man in the following couple was particularly good at expressing and owning the uncertainty he felt about how to improve his diet. Eighty pounds overweight, he was haunted by his failure to stay on one diet program and was "tired of being tired."

H: This affects you, but, I mean, this is *my* issue. You're really supportive of me when I do try. Now I just—I'm tired of trying. But I know I need to. I'm conflicted. I'm my own worst enemy in this. 'Cause I know I need to, but I don't *want* to.

W: Except it's *not* just your issue because if it's an issue that affects you, then it affects me, too. Don't feel like it's like something you've gotta, you know, do all by *yourself.*

Nice response! By being crystal clear in where he was in the process of making real changes, this man was able to evoke a compassionate and supportive response from his partner. In fact, she has given a textbook-quality statement of our first principle—the Principle of Mutual Influence—that lets her husband know *he is not alone.* He builds from there.

H: I lack self-discipline. I have difficulty controlling what I put into my body, and I'm very unmotivated to do things with my body to get it into shape. Not to mention I'm not the most honest when I'm doing it because I'm just not motivated to do it, which makes me feel even worse.

W: What can I say, sweetheart? I mean, I'm totally here to help you.

By honestly articulating his personal struggle without demanding any support, this man is informing his partner without putting any pressure on her to solve his problems. Though still a long way from his goals, he is effectively nurturing the support that he will need when he *is* ready to commit to a healthier way of eating.

MAKE IT EASY FOR YOUR PARTNER TO HELP YOU. The strong desire you have to eat right—even the desperation that you might be feeling about your weight or appearance—can be great if it drives you toward healthier eating. But intense feelings can just as easily drive away the help you need. We get overwhelmed emotionally when the changes we seek are too great, or too vague, or beyond our grasp. We become more difficult to understand and validate, and as a result the support our partner is able to offer will probably suffer. Most of us would rather support someone who has identified some clear, specific changes, and who has already shown a real commitment to making those changes. Statements like this one enable our partner to be effective and responsive:

> I'm not sure if you've noticed, but I took the dog for a walk both
> days last weekend, and I have stopped putting peanut butter on
> our toast in the mornings. I know these are just baby steps, but I
> just want to keep making small changes like this, stuff I know I can
> manage. Am I missing anything else obvious, stuff we wouldn't even
> notice?

ACCEPT INFLUENCE FROM YOUR PARTNER. When we're ambivalent about making a shift to healthier habits, we waffle. We say we want to change, but then we hold tight to what we know, as if the bad habits were a life preserver (*"You don't understand! My Pepsi's like cigarettes to me!"*). This is a natural reaction, but our partner's suggestions for better alternatives—the *real* life preservers—have to be considered and appreciated. Ultimately, this means you, the Waffler, need to find ways to accept your partner's influence.

We watched as one husband, feeling chubby and eating poorly because of demanding work and school schedules, strategized with his wife about one of his hardest problems: how to order the right foods in restaurants.

> **H:** You can prod me, I mean, I don't see it as nagging. Like, you know,
> "Oh, Mark, this salad looks *really* good! How about that?" Because
> otherwise I'll just go right for the hamburger without saying
> anything.
> **W:** Because that's not what I *believe* in. My feeling is you can eat just
> about whatever you want. You just don't have a huge portion.
> I mean, have that hamburger, but maybe if you've already had

146 LOVE ME SLENDER

enough calcium for the day, you don't have to have the slice of
cheese on it as well because the cheese is going to be fattening.
Or, you know, just don't get the french fries.

H: But then *say* that! Say, "You get the chicken on top of this pasta,
or else just get a burger, but with no bacon or cheese on it. Your
choice." You know? Then I'll say, "Hmm, I'm kind of hungry, I'd
rather have a chicken and pasta than a burger with nothing on it."

W: Or you can say, "Well, if I have this now, then tomorrow I'll have
a turkey sandwich with nonfat mayo on it."

H: And that's fine. I just don't see that as nagging. I don't see that
as you telling me what to do. I see it as you trying to *help* me
because, you know, you've got more expertise.

W: I would be more than happy to help you with that.

By welcoming his wife's suggestions rather than rejecting them—
"I just don't see that as nagging. . . . I see it as you trying to help *me"*—this
husband is making it easier for her to jump in with good support. He is
presenting a visible target to hit, actively cultivating the help he needs
to eat right and shed weight. Fully aware that they *influence* each other's
eating habits and choices, these two people are now building on that to
create the mutual *understanding* that will enable this husband to make
the right choices more often.

TAKE THE LEAD WHEN OFFERING NEW SOLUTIONS. Instead of holding up a tiny
moving target that you expect your partner to hit (*"What about spinach?"*;
"Nope, I hate spinach—but keep guessing!"), make your target bigger and
clearer (*"Hmm, spinach. Maybe. Or maybe I could try beets. Or zucchini"*).
Even better, stop waiting for your partner to solve the problem for you,
and instead suggest new ways of eating that you'd be willing to try.

If Your Partner Is a Waffler

If your partner consistently resists or rejects your suggestions for healthier eating, you may be misunderstanding what he or she really needs.

Listen hard to what your partner is saying, check to make sure you're on the right track, and connect with those feelings. But if your partner does seem to be a Waffler, the following strategies may help you understand and push through the sticking points:

ASSESS YOUR PARTNER'S READINESS TO CHANGE. There are legitimate concerns—excessive weight, fatigue, fear of clogged arteries, keeling over after chasing a toddler down the hall—motivating the Waffler's appeals for your help and support. But as tempting as it is for you to jump in with solutions the minute you hear your partner say "I need your help," doing so may be premature. A better tactic is to help your partner pinpoint these concerns and to then clarify whether they are sufficient motivation for real changes. The husband we introduced earlier, eighty pounds overweight and frustrated, could not have been clearer in expressing his main concern:

> **H:** My concern is, my problem is, I don't like being *tired*. I hate
> feeling like I can't go *do* something . . . But I mean, am I just
> not ready to change it? Because I get pretty fixated on this. But
> you know, I am doing it while I'm sitting on the couch, eating a
> peanut butter sandwich, watching TV or playing a video game.
> **W:** Are you tired because of lack of exercise, do you think, or eating
> poor foods, or both?
> **H:** Both.

By rushing in to identify some plausible solutions, this woman made the big mistake of assuming that her husband was ready to change. She asked a closed-ended multiple-choice question where she really needed an open-ended short essay. Better alternatives would involve drawing out the concerns (e.g., "*What sorts of things do you want to do but can't because you're too tired?*") and taking his question at face value (e.g., "*Well, I think you're asking the right question here. Have you thought about the possibility that you're just not quite ready to make this change? Once you set your mind to it, I am confident that you can eat better. But, do you feel you're ready?"*). Just because the Waffler's engine is running is no guarantee that he or she is actually in gear and ready to drive.

WORK WITH YOUR PARTNER TO OPEN UP THE RANGE OF OPTIONS. Even when their motivation is not in doubt, Wafflers are willing to consider only a limited set of solutions. Try not to take it personally, as this ambivalence reflects your partner's grappling with which new eating strategies he or she wants to adopt. Sidestep the "I propose/You oppose" Ping-Pong match by asking questions that *expand* your partner's options. Ask questions that encourage your partner to generate workable solutions of his or her own: *"Okay, so spinach isn't your thing. Have you thought about what kinds of healthier foods would work for you?"* Or, *"Okay, so you like to drink Pepsi in the afternoon, not so much because you like it but because it helps you to stay awake. So, can you maybe think of other, healthier ways to do that?"*

CLARIFY THE GROUND RULES. If your partner is a Waffler, sometimes the best approach is not so much to talk about the problem, but to talk about *how to talk about the problem.* This might sound like psychobabble, but clarifying the ground rules for conversations can reduce frustration and deepen understanding.

Remember that the Waffler is essentially saying, in perfect self-contradiction, *"I need your help, but I do not want your help."* Gently noting this disconnect can be a good way to sidestep this trap. For example, *"You know, on the one hand you are saying that you really do want to eat better and feel more energized, which I think is great. But then I see you snacking a lot. And when we talk about ways for you to eat better, you know, nothing seems to stick. I believe you when you say you want to eat healthier, but I guess I'm a bit confused about what it is I can do to help."*

Psychologists call these "process comments," and they are a powerful way to analyze a conversation that's not going the way it needs to go. One husband in our study was particularly good at drawing out this sort of self-contradiction.

W: Well, I'm not eating right. I've gained weight, I feel gross. I don't want to do things with your friends and stuff because I get embarrassed. I think they're going to look at me, talk, and, you know, say I've gained weight. And it makes me feel bad, because we could be doing more things and maybe I wouldn't feel so negative about myself . . . .

H: But if I tell you anything you just say, "What, are you calling me fat!?" And if I *don't* say anything, you say, "Why don't you ever *say* anything to me?"

This woman is struggling and wants her husband's help, and he stands by ready to deliver. But rather than take the bait and jump in with solutions, he says, in effect, "*I am a little confused about how best to help you, and I want you to help me to understand what you need here. Rather than me giving you solutions, which have not worked so well in the past, let's both work on figuring out the sorts of solutions that are likely to work best for you.*"

CHOOSE YOUR BATTLES WISELY. Being called a hypocrite is unsettling for most of us, highlighting as it does an uncomfortable gap between word ("*I'm committed to a lifetime of healthy eating*") and deed ("*As a matter of fact, I will have fries with that bacon cheeseburger*"). The anxiety that a Waffler feels is a product of this gap, and to cover it up he or she may resort to making excuses, minimizing health risks, or making extreme and even absurd comparisons. For example, upon learning that his wife did not have enough energy during the day, one husband suggested that she exercise and eat better. She then explained that she burned enough calories already by thinking.

Thinking burns calories. I do it for extended periods of time—hours and hours and hours. All day long. Think, think, think, think, think. That's physical energy. That's calories burned. It's significant.

This husband could argue with his wife about the effectiveness of thinking as a weight-management strategy, but he is better off agreeing and then refocusing on the real problem: "*I never really thought about it that way, but is thinking enough? I mean, maybe you could also eat healthier and get some exercise, too.*"

When one wife's husband complained that she was nagging him and restricting his diet too much, she called him a liar and proceeded to list all the foods she still allowed in the house: "*Those little Twinkie things, the chips you want, the Tostitos, the Doritos, the Toaster Strudels . . .*" He admitted, "*I know I need to eat better, but I could be so much worse. I mean, it's not like I sip down a twelve-pack of Pepsi a day and, you know, eat three sandwiches for lunch.*" Again, collusion may be the better response here, as there is little advantage to challenging the point: "*You're right, it could actually be much worse. Still, if you do want to eat* better, *where do you think you could start?*" Here it is best for her to see the smoke screen for the defense that it is, and to keep the focus on the bigger battle: healthy eating.

KEY POINTS FROM CHAPTER 5

- Often, partners can "set it and forget it" when they are already teaming up to eat healthy foods. But getting to this point, and remaining there, can be frustrating and emotionally demanding. Sometimes these emotions reflect personal vulnerabilities that are embarrassing or painful to express (*"I am unhappy with how I look and how much weight I have gained"*). At other times, the challenge to eat right can create emotional tension in the relationship. The other partner can feel threatened or criticized (*"Does this mean you find me unattractive now?"*).

- Mismanaged, these feelings and tensions will interfere with healthy eating. When partners collaborate as genuine allies, however, they tune in to these feelings. Doing so enables them to encourage and reinforce good dietary choices, while also supporting each other's efforts to eat right. This is the essence of our second principle, the Principle of Mutual Understanding.

- Applying the Principle of Mutual Understanding enables relationship partners to overcome *three common roadblocks in diet-related conversations.*

    In the first, the *Charmer* seems to be providing emotional support, while actually invalidating the partner's desires for healthier eating and weight loss, saying in effect, *"Don't change a thing! I think you look great!"*

    In the second, the *One-Trick Pony* offers reasonable advice about eating right but fails to recognize that the partner needs something entirely different: *"Here's what works for me! Just do it my way!"*

    In the third, the *Waffler* seeks the partner's support but then rejects it, saying, *"I really need your help to get my eating on the right track, but keep trying because every suggestion you offer will be inadequate!"*

- For each dilemma, appreciating the Principle of Mutual Understanding can help couples to identify several specific strategies that enable both partners to reach out, connect, and collaborate in their quest to eat right and slim down.

PLANNING FOR CHANGE

In this chapter, we have described a number of ways for couples to develop the mutual understanding that enables them to connect over diet and eating. Think about the level of mutual understanding between you and your partner right now. Each of the statements below describes something that successful couples do to support each partner's efforts to eat right. For each one, consider how well you and your partner engage in this behavior, and how easy or difficult it will be for the two of you to make any needed improvements.

1. We *recognize that we might be different* in how we want to eat better, how we want to be supported, and how we support each other.

    ____ This is a real strength for us. We do not need to make changes in this area.

    ____ We could improve in this area, and we think it will be easy to do so.

    ____ We could improve in this area, but we think it will be difficult to do so.

2. We *listen closely* to each other when one of us talks about how hard it is to eat right. We *pay attention to the emotions* we are expressing, and we *follow up with questions that open up or deepen our discussions* about healthy eating.

    ____ This is a real strength for us. We do not need to make changes in this area.

    ____ We could improve in this area, and we think it will be easy to do so.

    ____ We could improve in this area, but we think it will be difficult to do so.

3. We help each other to *clarify our specific goals* and diet-related improvements. We *team up to make these changes* part of our daily lives.

    ____ This is a real strength for us. We do not need to make changes in this area.

    ____ We could improve in this area, and we think it will be easy to do so.

    ____ We could improve in this area, but we think it will be difficult to do so.

4. We *ask for help and support* when we have a clear idea of what we need, and when we are ready to start making improvements in our diet.

    ____ This is a real strength for us. We do not need to make changes in this area.

    ____ We could improve in this area, and we think it will be easy to do so.

    ____ We could improve in this area, but we think it will be difficult to do so.

5. We *tailor our support to the specific changes* we are each trying to make to our diet. We pay attention to *how ready and motivated we both are* in the process of eating better.

____ This is a real strength for us. We do not need to make changes in this
area.

____ We could improve in this area, and we think it will be easy to do so.

____ We could improve in this area, but we think it will be difficult to do so.

6. We *express appreciation* for the support and encouragement that we give
each other when we are working to eat healthier. We emphasize what we
find most valuable in the support we receive.

____ This is a real strength for us. We do not need to make changes in this
area.

____ We could improve in this area, and we think it will be easy to do so.

____ We could improve in this area, but we think it will be difficult to do so.

7. We *avoid criticism* and insensitive comments about each other's eating habits and the support we exchange.

____ This is a real strength for us. We do not need to make changes in this
area.

____ We could improve in this area, and we think it will be easy to do so.

____ We could improve in this area, but we think it will be difficult to do so.

If you found yourself marking the first answer a lot, then you and
your partner clearly appreciate the Principle of Mutual Understanding
and have been exploiting that understanding to reinforce each other's
efforts to eat right.

If your responses tend toward the second answer, then you are well
on your way to real change. Now that you understand how the Principle of Mutual Understanding works, you and your partner have a
number of great ways to meet your goals for a healthier diet, and there
is nothing stopping you from working together to make those improvements happen.

If you found yourself often marking the third answer, then you and
your partner may grasp the Principle of Mutual Understanding but still
recognize that making this idea work for you in your own lives will not

be easy. This is to be expected; after all, eating right is hard by itself, and implementing this particular principle might put your communication skills to a real test. One way to get on track is to stay intently focused on the task at hand: exchanging high-quality support specifically in the domain of healthy eating. Try to avoid getting distracted by other challenges in your lives and in your relationship. Another way to get on track is to remember how much you and your partner share the long-term goal of getting healthy. Any quibbles you and your partner might have about eating right today might diminish when you appreciate how much you both want to live long and healthy lives. Our next chapter builds directly upon this point.

6

Eating Right and Long-Term Commitment

GETTING BEYOND THE DIET

"NOW THAT I'VE SEEN *the two extremes, I liked it the way I was before, and I want to go back.*" When Drew, an architect in his early forties, first came to our research rooms with his wife, Natalie, he seemed to know everything about diets. In fact, he'd been on *dozens* of them. Drew's expanding waistline annoyed him every time he looked in the mirror, spurring him into periodic fits of dieting. He tried cutting out bread and carbonated drinks. He tried going vegetarian. He tried skipping meals, eating smaller portions, drinking protein shakes, and consuming high-carb energy and granola bars. And all of these tactics worked—in the short term. He lost weight every single time. But then some crazy deadline kept him at work late for several nights in a row, or the kids got sick and neither he nor Natalie had time to cook. So, Drew found himself eating take-out cheeseburgers at his desk once again and, just like that, whichever diet he was on at the moment fell by the wayside.

It was a cycle going nowhere healthy, and Natalie was well aware of it. Despite being a dietitian, she found it extremely difficult to help Drew change his poor habits while balancing her job with the demands of raising two boys in elementary school. Natalie wanted to support her husband, but keeping him on task was a constant struggle. Watching him lose and gain the same thirty pounds over and over again pained her, and she was afraid of the serious illnesses that might lie in his future.

When they came to our lab to talk about their health, Natalie began by acknowledging the problem.

> **Natalie:** It seems to me that what happened was you lost weight and then you kind of slacked off. I mean, you stopped being as conscientious, you know? Instead of focusing on maintenance, you just go back into—
>
> **Drew:** *[interrupting]* But—
>
> **Natalie:** I mean, I know when we were on vacation we said we weren't going to worry about what we ate. And we said we would get back on track when we got home . . . But then, tonight you ordered the lasagna—
>
> **Drew:** *[interrupting]* I think now I realize that I got off track. I know the difference between approaching overweight—I mean being slightly overweight—and what I should be. Now that I've seen the two extremes, I liked it the way I was before, and I want to go back.

Natalie and Drew were on the right path, giving each other a chance to vent while acknowledging the need to change. When Natalie pointed out that Drew failed to return to his pre-vacation eating habits, he could have gotten defensive, but he didn't. Even though he was reluctant to admit just *how* overweight he had become, Drew knew that he had several pounds to shed. For her part, Natalie was concerned and involved. She recognized that she had an important role to play in getting Drew to watch what he ate; her professional training as a dietitian certainly helped when it came to deciding on which foods to buy and which ones to skip. But even though they'd both managed to have healthier diets in the past, Drew and Natalie couldn't find any solutions for the constant challenges of sticking to them.

> **Drew:** I was doing real well when I was back in Oregon, but then we moved down here and I took this new job . . .
>
> **Natalie:** *[enthusiastically]* You used to do real well! Remember when you were doing food diaries and stuff like that, and I was helping you, and you were a lot more conscious of what you put into your mouth?
>
> **Drew:** *[agreeing]* And then we moved down here and—I'm still conscious, it's just that I am starting to slack more. I just don't have any time! I think my schedule fluctuates too much. I would like to go back to what I was doing before.

Natalie's enthusiasm and support for her husband's efforts stemmed from genuine empathy. After all, she grappled with the same challenges.

> **Drew:** And what about your health? Pretty much fine?
>
> **Natalie:** Yeah. I mean, I would like to do the same thing. We just need to be more careful thinking about our meals, we need to make lists when we go to the grocery store, and I certainly could go out there and exercise more. This is the least that I've exercised in seven years.
>
> **Drew:** Well, in the last six months we were too busy helping with your sister's wedding.
>
> **Natalie:** You're right, but that should have been a motivation to eat better, not an excuse to slack off.
>
> **Drew:** It may have been a motivation, but there wasn't time! It's one thing to be motivated, but you can be motivated and not have any time to do anything about it.

Eating right takes time and effort, and to their credit Natalie and Drew both realized that. And they were both motivated to make that effort, and to work together as a team. But again and again, they ran into the same wall: no time to shop, no time to cook.

>   **Natalie:** Maybe you should start writing everything down again. You know, we put all that into that nutrition program and analyzed it. They're expensive, but I'm sure at work there's some other program I can find.
>
>   **Drew:** *[ignoring her suggestion]* Maybe we could also start planning a weekly menu. You know, like we are having stir-fry one night, we're having pasta one night . . .
>
>   **Natalie:** Don't you remember I did that last year? Like in May? That whole time we were cooking good stuff.
>
>   **Drew:** Oh, yeah.

The trajectory of their conversation, like the fluctuations in Drew's weight, is a roller-coaster ride. When Drew and Natalie returned to our research rooms two years later, Drew was quite a bit heavier than he had been at their first visit. Once again, a conversation about weight was on their agenda, and once again, Drew was embarking on a new diet.

>   **Drew:** Now that I am back to a regular work schedule, I have been getting in better health, eating salads and stuff and losing weight.
>
>   **Natalie:** I still think you need to try to learn portion control. Like today, when I told you that bowl was a serving bowl, not an eating bowl. I mean, you had a serving bowl full of Frosted Flakes.
>
>   **Drew:** Sure, but I didn't have breakfast, so . . .
>
>   **Natalie:** Still, it was a lot. I'm just saying.
>
>   **Drew:** Yeah, but I didn't have breakfast!
>
>   **Natalie:** And if we are out to eat, try to eat only half of your meal.
>
>   **Drew:** Half a meal? Then why order?
>
>   **Natalie:** Because restaurants give you way too much food.
>
>   **Drew:** I'm fine.

Natalie: I know you are. It's just something to work on. It's something
that has been a problem for a while, and we seem to have good
conversations about it, but we never put a plan into action. I just
want it to go somewhere this time and not just a lot of talk.

Only two years had passed since we first met this couple, but it
was obvious that their dynamic had changed quite a bit over that time.
Where Natalie had once been Drew's cheerleader, encouraging his
positive choices, now she had grown more critical, focusing on his missteps (*eating out of a serving bowl!*) and what she perceived to be his poor
choices (*cleaning his plate at restaurants!*). And where Drew had once been
open to Natalie's feedback, now he had grown more defensive ("*But I
didn't have breakfast!*"), rationalizing his tendency to order portions that
are larger than what's good for him. One gets the sense that these are
conversations that have repeated themselves with only minor variations
over their whole relationship.

The couples who talk about diet and nutrition in our research
rooms want to look good and feel better about themselves. Drew and
Natalie are several steps ahead of most of these couples because they
have already gotten over the highest hurdle—getting started. But Drew
and Natalie also prove that getting started, though necessary, is not sufficient. Losing weight and keeping it off require maintaining better eating
habits permanently. Many couples get stuck in this same kind of endless
loop—making resolutions, breaking them, and making them again—
repeating the exhausting trip from optimism to disappointment. How
can any of us break out of this discouraging pattern?

For couples who wrestle with staying on track with their diet and
eating habits, the Principle of Long-Term Commitment offers some
useful tools. According to this principle, our relationships are powerful because they can encourage us to remain mindful of our long-term
goals for better health even as we confront difficult choices about what
to eat in the here and now. In this chapter, we will discuss how we
can use the commitments we make to our partners to strengthen the

commitments we make to our own and to each other's health, and in so doing bolster our efforts to eat better. We will talk about what to do when our partner falls off the wagon, and about the three different traps they can fall into when they do. In each case, we will offer some suggestions for using the Principle of Long-Term Commitment to get out of these traps. But first we'll talk about the real reasons why dieting as most people practice it can be so mind-bogglingly hard.

FORGET ABOUT STICKING TO DIETS

The good news is that almost any diet that restricts calorie intake helps you lose weight. Researchers at Stanford University confirmed this in a 2007 study that randomly assigned more than 300 women to one of four popular diets based on best-selling books. No matter which diet they were assigned, the participants in the study lost an average of four to ten pounds in the first two months. Earlier reviews of research on dieting reached similar conclusions: most people who participate in a weight-loss program—any weight-loss program—can be expected to shed between 5 percent and 10 percent of their body weight.

The bad news is that the weight stays off only *while you are on the diet*. As soon as you come off of the diet, your old habits quickly resurface, and with them so does the weight. It's worse than just gaining back the lost pounds. One study found that within two years of ending their diets, more than 80 percent of dieters had gained back *more* weight than they lost. The longer former dieters are observed, the more weight they seem to gain over time, leading to an ironic and painful conclusion: for many people, dieting eventually makes you heavier. When it comes to eating habits, making a change that you cannot sustain may be worse than making no change at all.

Of course, some people do make changes that last. For about twenty years, the National Weight Control Registry at Brown University Medical School has studied more than 10,000 people who have lost significant amounts of weight and have kept it off. What do they all have in common? Not surprisingly, they are the ones who were able to adopt healthy eating habits and then make those habits an enduring part of their lives, in most cases drastically restricting their consumption of fat and their overall caloric intake for years at a time. Sounds good, but these people are rare—a tiny fraction compared with the millions of people whose efforts to control what they eat are much less successful. Those people, like Drew and Natalie, tell the far more familiar story of diets that work in the short term but never last.

Diets are not—and will never be—the sole answer to losing weight and keeping it off. As the people in the National Weight Control Registry understand, long-term weight maintenance requires permanent changes in eating habits—not quick-fix diets. Yet, as we pointed out in chapter 2, human beings are not especially adept at planning for the future; when you consider our evolutionary history, advances in public health have only recently given us a distant future to contemplate. Framed in this way, eating right comes down to answering one crucial question: *How can we fight against our tendencies toward short-term thinking and immediate gratification, and make the sustainable choices that can keep us eating healthfully, through to a healthy old age?*

Spoiler alert: It's not going to be easy. But instead of ignoring or denying that message, we are better off doing our best to embrace it and then mustering up the resources that will allow us to meet the challenge head-on. And this is where our relationships become crucial assets. The Principle of Long-Term Commitment suggests that we can use our commitment to our relationships to make eating right easier. The fact is that we are much more likely to sustain our commitments when we commit ourselves *to* something than when we commit ourselves *against* something. Positive goals (like having long and loving relationships) give us strength and drive us to overcome obstacles, whereas negative goals (like resisting that last slice of cake) require self-control and so become obstacles themselves.

Numerous studies show that when people keep their long-term

goals for a desired future in mind, they are more likely to make choices that serve those goals in the present. This is one reason why most people are far more successful at staying committed to their relationships than to their diets: in our relationships we naturally, and frequently, think about and plan for the future. When we do the same thing with respect to our eating habits—when we think about our long-term health and make specific plans for how to get there—studies show that we make better food choices and resist unhealthy snacks more effectively. But, as we have seen, that sort of thinking isn't second nature to us when we think about food. It is easy to look across the table at someone we love and imagine a long life with that person, but it is hard to stare at a plate of fries sitting on the same table and imagine a long life without them. *The trick, therefore, is to connect our choices about food to our goals for our relationships.* That is what the Principle of Long-Term Commitment can do for us. If we can link our desire to eat better to our desire for a good relationship, then eating better can be working toward something rather than fighting against something.

In the rest of this chapter, we show how applying this principle can help you and your partner avoid the pitfalls that keep us from making lasting changes to our eating habits. Couples in our research studies seem to face three kinds of obstacles here:

1. Facing the *Now-or-Never Problem,* some couples want to reach all their weight goals *right now* and find it difficult to stay motivated when they are not seeing steady results on the scale.

2. Some partners are *Dreamers,* setting goals that would be exceedingly hard for them to reach, and so have trouble finding the motivation to get started.

3. Finally, some couples get bogged down by the *Broken Egg Problem,* getting so frustrated when they do get off track with their eating habits that they give up completely, abandoning strategies that might well benefit them if given another chance.

As we describe each of these problems below, we will highlight how couples can take advantage of their commitment to each other to improve their chances of eating well on a regular basis.

"I HAVE TO SEE SOME KIND OF RESULT": THE NOW-OR-NEVER PROBLEM

No matter how diligently we watch what we eat, real weight loss takes time. As great as it would be to watch the pounds just magically melt away, our bodies simply don't work that way. Real change is usually incremental and happens in spurts. For some people, the lag between eating right and seeing results on the scale can be unbearable. And because they find changing lifelong eating habits painful in the short term, these dieters want a short-term payoff to justify their sacrifices. But they feel that steady but small changes are not significant enough. They want big results right away, and therefore lose steam when real weight loss is slow to come.

This is the *Now-or-Never Problem,* and people confront it whenever they are tempted to give up on eating better just because they have not yet seen the weight loss they are hoping to achieve. The wife in the following couple is a perfect example. An experienced dieter, she knows herself well enough to articulate why she has abandoned diets in the past, and why she is likely to abandon her current diet in the very near future.

> **W:** I know that in order for me to stick with anything, I have to see some kind of result. And that's my problem. Five years ago, I could just cut what I was eating in half, and by the end of the week I'd see a result. . . . I could just eat salad every day. I'd lose weight but I'd be very unhappy.
>
> **H:** That's the problem with all these diets.
>
> **W:** I'd be very cranky.

H: I remember a couple of weeks ago we were sticking to it pretty well, but all the food—I got so sick of eating the same food over and over again.

W: I know that consistency is my biggest problem. I can only say that I'm going to try, but part of the problem for me was I really felt like when I made the effort it didn't matter. If I'm not seeing a result, and if I'm seeing the *opposite* result, then what's the point?

This woman says that she is going to try to eat better, but already seems to be preparing for failure. She declares that she will make an effort to eat better only if a certain condition (i.e., "*seeing a result*") is met. Yet she knows that her chances of seeing that result are less now than they were five years ago. Without the promise of that result as an immediate reward, she can find no other compelling reasons to eat better.

Her husband might have offered some. He might have tried to motivate or encourage her, and to point out all the good reasons to eat healthy that go beyond immediate weight loss. But he does none of these things. Instead, he joins her in expressing pessimism and adds his own explanation for abandoning their plan ("*I got so sick of eating the same food over and over again*"). He *is* being supportive, true, but only of his wife's weaknesses—not the part of her that wants to be healthier.

Another husband took a harder line, but faced the same challenge. His wife had recently embarked on a drastic diet plan, cutting out major food groups and logging every bite in a detailed food diary. Several weeks into her plan, her weight loss had reached a plateau and tracking her meals became overwhelming. She was ready to give up, and looked to her husband for a lifeline. He tried to provide one.

H: I mean, everything just takes time. You can't lose ten pounds overnight.

W: I know, but I've been at this every day *hard core* for a month now.

H: But I think you believe that you can lose it overnight.

W: Well, I want to.

What she is actually expressing is a desperate need for some rein-forcement. She knows that without it, her current plan is ultimately unsustainable. Her husband understands. But in this conversation, he was unable to provide her with any substitute source of motivation that might have kept her going.

What these couples have in common is their focus on immediate experiences to the exclusion of everything else. They count the days until they can escape from eating plans that are making them miserable. For these couples, eating right is a means to an end—reaching their desired weight—so they treat changing their eating habits as a project to be completed as quickly as possible, rather than as a lifestyle they will have to maintain over time. This attitude—counting down the pounds and counting down the days—lies at the heart of the Now-or-Never Problem, and it makes the already difficult task of eating healthier a whole lot more frustrating.

The way out of the Now-or-Never Problem is to recognize that the bars of this cage are built from two faulty assumptions: 1) weight loss is praiseworthy only when it's quick; and 2) weight loss is the sole measure of health. Although saying so has become a cliché, it still bears repeating: Weight that takes years to gain may take years to lose, espe-cially if we plan to keep it off. In a world where living eighty years or longer is a real possibility, our plans to lose weight have to take decades into account, not weeks or months. And who says that weight loss is the only acceptable criterion for judging the success of a new diet? There are many other valuable reasons for making healthier food choices, in-cluding having more energy, staving off heart disease, and prolonging life. So, accepting these two assumptions uncritically leads to a kind of myopia; a relentless focus on the scale blinds dieters to the overarching goal of *better health,* a goal that should give meaning and purpose to the choices we make around food.

Yet, when day-to-day concerns about weight loom so large, adopting a broader perspective can seem impossible. That's where the Principle of Long-Term Commitment can help. By reminding us of the link between our individual well-being and our prospects for a long relationship, our partners can offer the additional motivation that some of us need to make eating well worthwhile. Thinking about our relationships can therefore help us break free of the narrow constraints of the Now-or-Never Problem.

If Your Partner Sees Weight Loss as "Now or Never"

If your partner is wrestling with the Now-or-Never Problem, understanding the Principle of Long-Term Commitment gives you several ways to be supportive (and if YOU are struggling with this problem, see if any of these solutions will help change your mindset):

ACKNOWLEDGE AND VALIDATE THE FRUSTRATION. Impatience is the hallmark of the Now-or-Never Problem. You can almost imagine the wife we described earlier throwing up her hands as she asks, "*What's the point?*" and you can surely hear the hint of a whine when our other example explains, "*but I've been at this every day* hard core *for a month now.*" These are the powerful feelings that defeat even our best intentions to make new eating habits last, and we ignore them at our own peril.

Try this instead: when frustration rises up and threatens to derail progress, recognize these feelings and help your partner to see them as a natural part of attempting something difficult. Just as we don't walk away from our partners the moment they refuse to relinquish the remote or to make some other compromise, we can't abandon our plans for healthy eating the moment those plans prove challenging. Of course it's challenging! For many people, we are talking about changing the habits of a lifetime.

The wife in the following example does a great job making this point. Her husband, another serial dieter, was in our research rooms beating himself up about his failure to stick to his latest diet. She could have browbeaten him, changed the subject, or told him to "just think positive," but instead she says:

> I know that the way we have our lifestyle arranged right now does not really cater real well to dieting because we eat out a lot. We celebrate with food, and we get depressed with food, and we— whatever—we eat when we're bored. We do all these things with food, and that's not conducive to eating right. But, you know, this does need an immediate solution because it's going to make you feel better if you can start doing it. And I want you to feel better and to stop feeling so bad about it.

She does two things skillfully here. On the one hand, her message is that the difficulties her husband is facing are natural and reasonable, given their circumstances. She understands his feelings and validates them, and that is likely to reinforce his sense that she is on his side. On the other hand, she does not allow those feelings to let him off the hook. The combined message is: 1) yes, you have the perfect right to feel frustrated; and 2) let's work together to find a way forward anyway. Where this woman might have treated her husband's frustration as an excuse to give up, she instead views it as a signal to get serious.

FOCUS ON LONG-TERM GOALS. Eating right will hold little appeal for your partner if it means giving up everything sweet and crispy—or whatever else he or she thinks is tasty. When your partner is mired in the Now-or-Never Problem, those sacrifices are all that he or she can see. Drawing on the Principle of Long-Term Commitment, you can remind your partner of the long-term goals that those sacrifices are serving. If eating right is less about resisting temptation and more about living longer, having more energy, and preserving your relationship far into old age, then a commitment to eating right is just a small slice of a larger commitment to the relationship. That is a commitment your partner has already made, and a powerful source of motivation when other rewards are lacking.

The following couple, both in their early twenties, spent most of their time in our research rooms discussing her fears that her efforts to lose weight weren't having much effect. To keep her motivated, this husband declared that he would join her in a weight-loss program, and here he explained why.

> **H:** I want to be in the best shape of my life too so I can last for you, you know?
> **W:** Aw, that's sweet!
> **H:** We're getting old. And you know, I want to be able to carry you.
> **W:** You want to be old and be in shape.
> **H:** Yeah, that's right. Old and strong and carry you across the threshold at seventy-five like, *[grunting]* "Rarh! Strong man, strong man!"

Look at the excitement that eating right can inspire! This husband is having so much fun playing with the image of himself as a healthy old person. It is easy to imagine his infectious enthusiasm for their shared future eventually brightening her attitude in the present.

For many of the couples we have studied, dreams of the parents they hope to be offer still another long-term goal. The following husband, recently married and raising two children from a previous relationship, was particularly eloquent as he described to his new wife how his goals as a father inspire his desire to eat better.

> I just feel like—I know if I can be a little healthier, stick to my food groups and stuff, I'll be in better shape, you know? And I'm not trying to get in shape to impress anybody, but I want to be in shape for you and I want to be healthy and I want to live longer. I see all these older people that are always complaining about this, complaining about that, and it's like, man, if that's what I'm looking forward to when I get older, I don't want that. I want to be able to grow up with my kids healthy and keep up with them. I want to

be able to take my son to play tennis or racquetball or go running or whatever and whip his ass at it, you know? I want to be able to go up against my son and show him what's up. And you know, my daughter is going to be sixteen, I'm going to be fifty-six. I want to be able to keep up with her. I want to be a little healthier and set a good example for the kids. You know, a healthy life, and a healthy relationship, too.

When this husband sits down to dinner with his family, he dreams about being a strong, active dad for his children rather than focusing on all the foods he is not eating. That's a much prettier picture, and it casts his food choices in a different light.

ENJOY THE PROCESS. When our partners are mired in the Now-or-Never Problem, the world of healthy eating feels devoid of pleasure. Their complaints about dieting are really cries for something—anything!—that feels like a reward for all their work. But the only rewards they can imagine involve the very foods that they are struggling to avoid. No one can be expected to live this way for long.

We can help our desperate partners by giving them what they are asking for, that is, by making eating right less bleak and more fun. Research by Daniel Ariely, a behavioral economist at Duke University, shows that we are more likely to persist at tasks that require self-control when we pair them with things that we naturally enjoy. Your relationship with your partner can provide that necessary pleasure.

A little creativity goes a long way here. Your partner doesn't like healthy foods like spinach? Maybe those greens will seem more appealing if they are the spoils of a weekly stroll together through your local farmers' market. Your partner skips breakfast? Hand her a pack of sliced apples or a strawberry-yogurt smoothie as she heads out the door. Diet plan getting boring? We know of one couple that competes to see who can make the tastiest vegetables for their kids. And don't underestimate the power of praise. If you take note and offer a compliment whenever your partner resists temptation (*"I know you could have ordered the spaghetti carbonara, but you ordered the chicken breast instead. You rock!"*), you are offering a powerful and immediate reward that no one else can provide. Sometimes a little recognition can make a lot of difference.

"I JUST WANT TO LOOK LIKE
A SUPERMODEL": THE DREAMER

Many of us talk about weight loss the same way we talk about the lottery. Asked what you would do with a winning ticket, you'd probably make a lengthy list of ridiculously expensive things to buy and daydream about your glitzy life as a new millionaire. Nevertheless, the fact that you can so vividly imagine a life of great wealth does not mean that you think about paying the property taxes on your new mansion, or paying insurance on your new Bentley. Some people have similarly lofty ambitions for their own figure. They can tell you exactly how they want to look, how amazing it would feel to look that way, and the new clothes they already have picked out. But they never get around to developing a plan that might bring their extravagant goals within reach. This is the pattern of the *Dreamer*. He or she sets unrealistic goals and then uses the unlikeliness of reaching them as an excuse to avoid getting started.

Part of us wants our partners to be Dreamers. After all, we want our partners to have big goals, especially when it comes to their health. What could be wrong about wanting to be fit and gorgeous? The problem with Dreamers is not that they want to lose weight, but that their desires are disconnected from any actions that contribute to weight loss—and often times, they set unrealistic goals that actually impede their weight-loss efforts. Ask yourself to lose ten pounds, and you can begin taking steps to make that happen, but ask yourself to look like Keira Knightley or Ryan Gosling, and you can only dream of having enough money to hire a personal chef and a full-time trainer. What looks at first like ambition turns out to be a strategy—even if an unconscious one—to avoid committing to real change.

How do you know whether your partner (or you) is serious about losing weight or is actually a Dreamer? There are a couple of telltale signs. First, people who are serious about getting healthier compare themselves with imagined future selves, and use the distance between the two as a source of inspiration (e.g., "*My goal is to weigh thirty pounds less than I do now*"). Dreamers, in contrast, imagine themselves looking like others, often others who look nothing like them. Now the distance is too wide to cross, and so the Dreamer does nothing. Several pounds above where she wants to be, the wife in the following example is this sort of Dreamer. In our research rooms, she spent her time talking with her husband about how it made her feel to go out with her girlfriends the previous weekend. She found that kind of socializing extremely threatening.

> **W:** We saw these really skinny, skinny girls. Meanwhile, I'm next to
> Pammy, who's five feet tall and like a size negative five. And all
> these girls are in these leather pants. And I'm like "Oh. My. God."
> I want to look like that.
> **H:** So you want to wear leather pants? That's something I needed to
> know before we got married!
> **W:** *[not laughing]* You *know* what I mean!

What *does* she mean? Does she mean that Pammy's and the other girls' leather pants are an inspiration that motivates her to give up between-meal snacks and make a real effort to eat right? Unlikely. She means that fitting into those pants is so far from where she sees herself now that thinking about what it would take to get there makes her feel helpless. Her dreams of looking like Pammy are not an inspiration but a source of anxiety. Instead of talking about the gradual weight loss that could lead to better health and a slimmer figure, Dreamers let their envy quash the subject altogether.

This leads us to our second point. People who are serious about getting healthier appreciate that losing weight means *taking action*. They

focus on their goals and on how they are going to reach those goals, defining the specific changes they are going to have to make in how they
eat. The Dreamer, in contrast, wants to lose weight, but rejects the idea
that doing so will require any substantive actions or sacrifices. This next
husband is this sort of Dreamer.

W: Why do you think you eat the way you eat?

H: Because I just like food. It's not emotional. It's definitely not
emotional. It's a problem because I'm gaining weight. That's the
only problem. But if I could eat and not gain weight I wouldn't
have a problem with it. We wouldn't even be talking about this
right now . . . I mean, you being supportive is not the issue
because you've basically been supportive of everything I've been
trying to do. It's just me being disciplined. There's just too much
good food out there.

W: Great food.

H: And I don't ever want to break the relationship between me and
food.

W: I know. I don't want to break that relationship either.

H: You know, cheeseburgers, my favorite. My babyback ribs. Anything
with potatoes.

W: Anything with butter . . .

H: Ahhh, butter.

This husband recognizes that his recent weight gain is a problem,
and he clearly would like to weigh less. At the same time, he loves the
way he eats right now, and seems to feel entitled to eat whatever he
wants, as much as he wants (e.g., "*I don't ever want to break the relationship
between me and food*"). You might expect that the conflict between these
two desires would cause him some tension. It does for many people,
who then become motivated to find ways to resolve the tension—
either by changing what they eat or by abandoning their goals. But this
husband resolves the tension another way: by fantasizing that he can get

everything he wants ("*If I could eat and not gain weight I wouldn't have a problem with it*"). Most people recognize this very common fantasy for what it is, and then move past it to face reality. Not the Dreamer.

For the Dreamer, the fantasy serves an important function: it is a way of quieting the part of him that knows he ought to make a change in his lifestyle. The moment this husband acknowledges that he has a problem ("*I'm gaining weight*"), he immediately starts to daydream about a world where he could be thin while still eating all the ribs, cheeseburgers, and buttery potatoes that he wants. Thinking of these things makes him feel better, lessening any tension that might need to be resolved through action. Peter Gollwitzer, a professor of psychology at New York University, calls this *premature consumption,* and it happens whenever daydreaming about reaching a goal gets in the way of taking steps toward that goal. When we fantasize, life seems to be a bit more vivid and bright—unrealistically so. We think about our goals in glowing terms, but that same glow blinds us to the difficult steps we will need to take to actually achieve those goals, reducing our motivation.

At the heart of the Dreamer's problems lies misunderstanding of the Principle of Long-Term Commitment. Dreamers often look like people who are committed to their long-term goals—and they certainly talk about them often enough. However, real long-term commitment involves being dedicated to a desired outcome and to *the process of achieving that outcome.* Dreamers skip right over that process, and so their repeated claims of wanting to weigh less are themselves weightless.

If Your Partner Is a Dreamer

If your partner is a Dreamer, the best support you can offer is a reminder of what commitment really means, and to help your partner make that same level of commitment to his or her health. Drawing upon the Principle of Long-Term Commitment, here are a few specific ways to help translate your partner's fantasies into reality (and if YOU are the Dreamer, see if these strategies change your perspective):

BRING YOUR PARTNER TO EARTH, GENTLY. If your partner is proposing a goal that he or she can't reach, then you do your partner no favors by following him or her into a fantasy. Instead, a loving partner can help focus the Dreamer on attainable goals, as a prerequisite for a discussion of how to reach those goals.

Navigating these waters can be tricky. You do not want to scold but you need to be firm, and that is a delicate balance. Look again at the conversation with the husband who wanted to eat ribs and potatoes and never gain weight. When he expressed this impossible wish, his wife followed along, echoing his rapturous descriptions of the foods he loves. Without entirely raining on his parade, she could have grounded her husband by saying something like this:

> Of course you want to eat and not gain weight! So do I! And I know
> that eating great food is important to you. It's important to me, too.
> Still, until they invent a magic pill, we are going to have to face the
> fact that we can't do everything we want to do forever. Your health is
> nonnegotiable. I need you to stick around for a long time. And that
> means something is going to have to change. So what do you really
> want to do about your weight? How are we going to know when
> you've met your goal?

Look at all that this sort of statement can accomplish. In the same breath, you can recognize the appeal of your partner's fantasies, acknowledge that you share them, *and* redirect the conversation back toward reality. By asking some pointed questions, this wife encourages her husband to describe realistic goals, without imposing any particular ones on him.

LINK LONG-TERM GOALS FOR THE FUTURE TO CONCRETE BEHAVIORS IN THE PRESENT. An ambitious goal can inspire us to great heights, as long as it accompanies explicit steps for reaching that goal. The Dreamer skips over those steps but you can shine a light on them, focusing your partner's attention on specific ways to change his or her diet *today*.

Imagine if the wife who wanted to fit into those leather pants had a partner who took this approach. When she shared how threatened she felt after going out with her much skinnier friends, her husband made a joke. If he had instead taken her disclosure seriously, when she exclaimed, *"You* know *what I mean!"* he might have responded with something like this:

> Honey, I do know what you mean. I know where you want to be
> with your weight, and I know that it tears you up when you feel like
> it would be impossible for you to get there. It tears *me* up to see you
> feeling so helpless. But here's the thing: you *can* get there. It's not like
> you have to become vegetarian or something overnight, but there are
> steps you can take that will make a real difference, and I am totally
> ready to take them with you. Like, just ordering take-out less often
> would be a big step. I know we are both really busy with work and
> the kids, but what if we reserved one night a week for cooking at
> home? Like maybe Sundays? I would love to do that with you, and
> the bonus is that we'll have leftovers for the rest of the week if we
> plan it right. Sure, it's a little step, but the weeks add up. It gets us
> started, that's the important thing, and I bet there are other changes
> we can make too.

Statements like these bring the Dreamer back to the daily life that the two of you share, and that is where you have to take the first steps toward eating better. Stay focused on finding solutions in the choices the two of you make every day.

FOCUS ON CHANGES YOU CAN MAKE PERMANENT. It's easy to propose strict food guidelines, but it's almost impossible to stick to them for long. Give up french fries forever? Eliminate all desserts? What a great way to make a long life sound awful. So don't bother considering changes that you already know your partner cannot or will not sustain. Instead, help your partner to identify ways of improving his or her diet that can realistically be woven into the fabric of your lives—not as a temporary measure but as a new way of living. Eliminating french fries and desserts forever may be impractical, but cutting back on them forever is not.

When we saw her in our research rooms, the wife in the following couple was heartbreakingly clear about her inability to resist sweets. She was on the verge of giving up entirely. Listen to how her husband used what we suggest above to pull her back from the brink.

W: I know that I can't do like I've always done over the years and think, "Well, I'm going to just whip myself into shape and write myself a diet and just go by it and stick to it." I'm to the place now where I'm being realistic. I'm not going to all of a sudden, overnight, be eating salads and fresh meat and fresh vegetables. I don't have any willpower when it comes to the sweets. I just don't have any willpower. If I haven't kept my blood sugar right or something, I'll start craving sweets like they're cocaine.

H: Okay, but I think—I feel like there should be some small little areas that we could start with that would be within your grasp. Remember what that one book said? Just concentrate on two things at a time. Like, you know all those menus I tack up on the refrigerator? Instead of trying to say that every night we're going to have some healthy planned meal, maybe we could start off with just one night a week when we're going to have the two vegetables and the main entrée and the salad. Just start off with one or two nights a week maybe. With our kind of hectic schedule, doesn't that feel more reachable?

If this husband had insisted that his wife stick to a rigid set of rules, he would have guaranteed her another demoralizing failure. Instead he takes a different approach, giving her options that represent a manageable change to the lifestyle they already share. Where her own thoughts leapt to dietary restrictions she knew she could not maintain, her husband gave her realistic goals that were well within her grasp. A success with the smaller changes her husband has proposed may be an important step toward continuing healthy changes in the future.

"BUT I TRIED THAT ALREADY!": THE BROKEN EGG PROBLEM

When success at losing weight is defined as following inflexible food rules, failure is inevitable. We all have to eat. Healthy and unhealthy foods surround us in our homes, at work, and on the road. Getting through a day, therefore, requires a nearly constant stream of choices about what to put into our mouths and what to avoid. The recommended healthy options aren't always available, and even when they are, no one reaches for the tofu and steamed broccoli every time. So any resolutions we make about eating right—No more carbs! No more desserts! Only home-cooked meals!—should come with a disclaimer: This resolution absolutely, positively will be broken.

The difference between people who do lose weight and people who don't lies in what happens next. Remember Drew and Natalie, the couple who had tried one diet after another, never managing to stick to any of them for very long? Consistency was their problem, but what they did have going for them was *persistence*. They never gave up and remained hopeful that the next program would be the one that helped them to lose weight and keep it off. Drew and Natalie kept alive their chances of finding dieting options they could make permanent. Not every couple has the stamina to maintain that optimism. For some people, failing to stick to a diet feels so bad that afterward they cannot imagine climbing back on that horse and trying again. This is the *Broken Egg Problem*. For those who suffer from it, one slipup is disaster from which there can be no recovery. As a result, they shortchange themselves, abandoning potentially beneficial strategies too soon.

As hard as it can be for anyone to shift toward healthier eating habits, the Broken Egg Problem makes it harder by giving serial dieters one more burden to bear: shame over their own perceived weakness. When a plan to eat better doesn't work or doesn't last, dieters can make excuses by blaming their circumstances (e.g., *"I could have done it, but it was a really busy time at the office."*) or blaming the plan itself (e.g., *"I should have known that* [insert fad diet here] *was a sham."*). However, those suffering from the Broken Egg Problem blame *themselves.* They underestimate how remarkably difficult it can be to eat right. And instead of redoubling their efforts or getting support, they interpret their failure to maintain a diet plan as a sign that they may not have had the ability to reach their desired weight in the first place. The stakes for their self-image are high, making the prospect of trying to lose weight again—already an emotionally sensitive issue—even more terrifying. Victims of the Broken Egg Problem can't go forward, for fear of confronting their limitations on yet another new diet. But they can't go back either because weight-loss plans that failed in the past are bound to trigger feelings of guilt.

One husband in our research rooms was especially articulate about this experience. A middle-school administrator with three young children, he had been troubled by his excessive weight for years. When he and his wife discussed his health in our research rooms, he explained why he was feeling so helpless.

I usually end up beating myself up over it, but it is my problem, and I don't know if I can expect a solution. I mean, I am essentially sixty pounds overweight for my height, for who I am supposed to be. And sixty pounds is just so daunting. And I mean, I felt like I was doing really good with the Body for Life, but I don't know. I was running every day, and I was trying with limited success to control what I was eating. But then you know, I hurt my back at work and I kind of dropped the ball. And now I feel like I've done Body for Life, and

I failed at it, so I don't feel like I can get back into it. I'm just—I'm tired of trying. I'm my own worst enemy in this. Because I failed at it, and I'm scared of failing again.

Being sixty pounds overweight would be daunting for anyone, but this husband has a second problem that makes it even more daunting: the memory of his failure to lose the weight the last time around. As we have discussed before, eating right is hard for so many reasons, yet look who this husband sees as his real enemy: himself! The blend of anxiety about his weight and disappointment in himself makes a toxic cocktail that can impede his chances of meeting his goals in the future, contributing to the cycle of helplessness and shame.

Like the Now-or-Never Problem and the Dreamer, the Broken Egg Problem arises from a misunderstanding of the Principle of Long-Term Commitment. The husband in our example certainly believes that he is committed to losing weight. In fact, he might say that his initial commitment is the reason he feels so terrible each time that he fails in his efforts to control what he eats. What he misses, however, is that the *purpose* of commitment is to get us back on our feet. We commit to things like losing weight (or saving for retirement or writing a book) so that we will persist through the inevitable rough spots. People who suffer from the Broken Egg Problem treat eating right as a test that they can't retake if they fail. Given that everyone will fail at some time or another, this is not a very useful strategy. Eating right is not like taking a test; it's like . . . well, it's like being in a relationship.

Recognizing the similarity between our commitments to our partners and our commitments to our health is the key to escaping the Broken Egg Problem. Our relationships with our partners are not over each time we misunderstand or disappoint each other. Why not? Because people fall short in relationships all the time, and we accept that. When we share a life with another person, we know that there will be stumbles and fights. We also know that couples can make up, resolve their disagreements, and continue their journeys together. That capacity for adjustment, compromise, and forgiveness turns out to be an excellent model to guide our lifelong pursuit of good health as well.

If Your Partner Is Experiencing the Broken Egg Problem

If your partner is having trouble recovering from a slipup and you suspect that the Broken Egg Problem has taken hold, there are several ways that you can get your partner beyond self-blame and back to making healthy choices (and if YOU are the one suffering from this problem, read on to find some solutions for yourself, too):

MODEL FORGIVENESS. When your partner is despondent over eating that third slice of pizza, it does no good to pile on more criticism. Instead, help your partner see that, in the context of a long-term commitment to eating right, one night's overindulgence is not that bad, and is certainly no reason to give up entirely. The wife of the husband in our previous example understood this. After her husband expressed his shame over having abandoned his previous diet plan, she responded by placing his behavior in perspective.

> It's not just your issue. Because it's an issue that affects you, it affects me. So don't feel like it's like something you have got to do all by yourself. And as far as "failing" at Body for Life, it's Body for *Life*. How many more years do you have left on your life? You have your whole life ahead of you to do this.

With these words, she reinforced her support for her husband's struggles with weight loss, and she provided something else that he desperately needed: the space to make mistakes.

APPRECIATE SMALL VICTORIES. Through the lens of the Broken Egg Problem, your partner sees only success on one side and failure on the other when it comes to dieting. You can help your partner reject this false dichotomy and appreciate the real achievements that lie between those extremes. When our partners are worried that all their efforts to eat better amount to nothing, they need us to remind them of what they have accomplished already, and could still accomplish with continued effort.

The husband in the following example took this approach with his wife, who looked back on all the diets she had tried in the past and saw only a string of failures. She was ready to give up trying, but her husband offered a different interpretation:

H: I think you're actually good at it when you set your mind to it.

W: Yeah?

H: Remember last year? That's probably the second most proud I've been of you.

W: *[laughing]* 'Cause I lost weight?

H: No, because you stuck with it.

W: Yeah, it took forever, though.

H: The Atkins, you tried that, but you didn't do it that well . . . but the Weight Watchers—you went to the meetings and you did it. And it worked and you felt good about yourself, so that's probably the happiest I've been with you other than when you had the baby.

The image that our partner holds of him- or herself is heavily influenced by what we think and say. This husband understands this, so when his wife sees herself as a failure, he holds a mirror up to her successes and the pride he takes in them. True, the weight loss she achieved last year did not last. But by focusing on the fact that she actually did lose weight when she tried, he reminds her of her capacity to change her habits, and he gives her the strength to try again.

TRY SOMETHING NEW. Something that eggs and diet plans have in common is that both are cheap and easy to find. Breaking an egg doesn't mean swearing off eggs; another one is usually within reach. The same is true for healthy diets. If one strategy turns out not to fit within your lifestyle, then another one might. One wife, a veteran of numerous diets, had been doubtful about a new plan, thinking it would be no different from the old ones they had tried. Her husband gave her confidence a boost by emphasizing the novelty of the latest changes they had made to the way they ate.

> We have to continue what we started last week. We've been doing
> it for the past two weeks and I want it to continue. I want it to be a
> regular part of our lives—and certainly my life, for sure. I mean, I will
> never ever, ever, *ever* in my entire life ever give up my passion for ribs
> and Mexican food. At the same time, I want us both to have better
> eating habits. I like the fact that we're eating more low-fat kind of
> stuff and I like the fact that we're eating several small meals a day
> instead of one or two really large ones. I hate skipping meals all day
> long, and I'm glad we're changing that, and I want it to continue.

This does not sound like just another diet, for a few reasons. First, this husband recognizes that the changes they are making need to become *a regular part of our lives* and not just temporary measures. Second, he understands that there is room for flexibility in their plan: eating *more low-fat kind of stuff* does not mean he has to give up his *passion for ribs and Mexican food*. Finally, he lets his wife know that, if one plan for eating right is not working out (*skipping meals all day long*), it is okay to try something new (*several small meals a day*). All of this reflects a long-term commitment to eating right, and improves the chances that this couple will maintain that commitment.

KEY POINTS FROM CHAPTER 6

- Losing weight and keeping it off require more than just getting started on eating right; they require making permanent changes to what we eat. Those changes can be hard to sustain when our bodies and our psychological makeups seem designed to resist weight loss.

- Although it is hard to make long-term plans when it comes to food, it is natural to think long-term when it comes to our relationships. Connecting our choices about food to our goals for our relationships makes eating right a step toward a long life with our partners, instead of another sacrifice.

- Exploiting the long-term perspective that commitment to our relationships provides gives us the tools we need to help our partners sidestep three common barriers to making lasting changes in the foods they eat.

- When our partners are impatient, demanding immediate results and growing frustrated when they are not forthcoming (*the Now-or-Never Problem*), we can use their aspirations for the relationship to remind them of all the good reasons to eat right that go beyond weight loss.

- When our partners are unrealistic, setting impossible goals that leave them feeling overwhelmed and helpless (*the Dreamer*), we can focus their attention on small, manageable changes that can have a big impact on weight when accumulated over a long life together.

- When our partners are rigid, abandoning promising strategies for eating right after each lapse in self-control (*the Broken Egg Problem*), we can offer perspective, appreciating their accomplishments and encouraging them to continue working toward the goals for health that the two of you share.

PLANNING FOR CHANGE

This section invites you to think about how you and your partner are exploiting your long-term commitment right now. Each of the statements below describes something that successful couples do to sustain each partner's efforts to eat right. For each one, consider how well you and your partner engage in this behavior, and how easy or difficult it will be for the two of you to make any needed improvements.

1. We *recognize and validate each other's feelings* about how hard it can be to eat right and lose weight.

   ____ This is a real strength for us. We do not need to make changes in this area.

   ____ We could improve in this area, and we think it will be easy to do so.

   ____ We could improve in this area, but we think it will be difficult to do so.

2. We remind each other that *making healthy food choices supports our long-term goals* for our relationship.

   ____ This is a real strength for us. We do not need to make changes in this area.

   ____ We could improve in this area, and we think it will be easy to do so.

   ____ We could improve in this area, but we think it will be difficult to do so.

3. We think about ways to *make the process of eating right fun and enjoyable*.

   ____ This is a real strength for us. We do not need to make changes in this area.

   ____ We could improve in this area, and we think it will be easy to do so.

   ____ We could improve in this area, but we think it will be difficult to do so.

4. We *set realistic goals* for weight loss and *consider how we will achieve* those goals.

   ____ This is a real strength for us. We do not need to make changes in this area.

   ____ We could improve in this area, and we think it will be easy to do so.

   ____ We could improve in this area, but we think it will be difficult to do so.

5. We *forgive ourselves and each other* when we fail to exercise self-control over what we eat.

_____ This is a real strength for us. We do not need to make changes in this area.

_____ We could improve in this area, and we think it will be easy to do so.

_____ We could improve in this area, but we think it will be difficult to do so.

If you found yourself marking the first answer a lot, then you and your partner clearly appreciate the Principle of Long-Term Commitment and have been exploiting that commitment to reinforce each other's efforts to eat right.

If your responses tend toward the second answer, then you are on your way. Now that you understand how the Principle of Long-Term Commitment works, you and your partner have a number of great ways to keep each other on track, and there is nothing stopping you from working together to make eating healthier a permanent part of your lives.

If you found yourself often marking the third answer, then you and your partner may understand the Principle of Long-Term Commitment but still recognize that making that commitment work for you in your own lives will not be easy. Consider reviewing this chapter again with an eye toward identifying concrete steps that you can take today. Remember that any frustrations you have experienced in the past should not register as failures as much as they are a reminder that you need a new and better strategy. You hold the key to converting your partner's long-term goals into healthy sacrifices that he or she will want to make today, and with your invitation your partner can do the same for you. Allow small successes to accumulate, and build from there.

PART III

TEAMING UP
TO MOVE MORE

JUST DO IT? JUST DUET.

By now, most people know that a long and healthy life means getting or staying fit. All the couples we have described so far share these goals, and if you are reading this book, you probably share them too. In the previous three chapters, we focused on one path to fitness—eating right—but that is not a path that works for everyone. Luckily there is another strategy that is just as powerful: getting active. In Part III, we'll show how the same three principles we discussed in Part II to help us eat right can also be harnessed to help us achieve another fitness goal: moving more.

7

Moving More and Mutual Influence

GETTING YOUR MOVE ON—TOGETHER

REG AND RITA, a young couple in their late twenties, were excitedly preparing for the birth of their first child. Along with registering at Babies "R" Us and taking Lamaze classes, they were thinking about their health. They had read all the parenting books and they knew that having kids, with all the joy it brings, does not leave parents with a lot of time to take care of themselves. Already dissatisfied with their weight, Greg and Rita were especially motivated to avoid additional weight gain that might set them up for health problems down the road.

They agreed that their problem was their jobs (he sold life insurance, she ran a doctor's office), which kept them behind desks and on the telephone a lot of the time. Quitting was not an option, so they knew the answer had to be exercise. They needed to get more active and burn some calories, but this was something they had been repeating to each other for a while with little to show for it. With the baby coming, it was finally time to figure out how to incorporate exercise into their lives, before the chaos of parenthood made real change even more difficult.

When they visited our research rooms, Greg and Rita chose to talk about developing a plan for being more active. But somehow, even though both of them *knew* they needed to exercise more, and even though both of them *wanted* to exercise more, the conversation we observed did not get them any closer to a plan for making it happen. On the contrary, the more they talked, the less likely it seemed that they would be able to develop the plan they wanted.

> **Rita:** *[whining]* I want to be skinny.
> **Greg:** *[laughs]* That's the issue we've had the most problems with, huh?
> **Rita:** Yeah . . .
> **Greg:** I know you want to do something about it and—
> **Rita:** We need to light a fire under each other's tails. I need you to motivate me and you need me to motivate you. I especially want to do something about it after the baby is born. Just like you don't want to be a big dad, I don't want to be a big mom. I want to make sure that we start exercising more. But before we get into it, I don't want you lecturing me. I'd like to start walking, and to make it a daily routine. I want to make sure we do it together as a team.

Rita has the right idea: she recognizes that each of them can help the other one move more, and that there are clear benefits if they can coordinate their efforts. But a mere twenty-five seconds into their conversation, there are signs of the tensions that are going to make this difficult. As she expresses her commitment to teamwork, Rita also conveys her reluctance to trust Greg as a true collaborator, first by warning him about his tendency to lecture her (before he has even finished a sentence), and second by announcing a plan for a new walking routine (without inviting his feedback or input). The mixed message is not lost on Greg.

> **Greg:** Let me ask you something as we're sitting here. I don't think that's fair to say, "Before you start lecturing." You just said that a second ago and it really hurts me.

Rita: Well, I can tell by the look in your eyes that you were getting ready to let me have it.

Greg: I wasn't going to lecture you and I don't think I do lecture you. I just tell it like it is. And all I was going to tell you was that it takes your own personal motivation, and here you are saying that I've got to motivate you and you've got to motivate me. Deep down, you get mad when I try to kick you in the butt.

Greg and Rita intended for this to be a conversation about how they are going to exercise more—a goal they share—but it has become something else: an argument over whose fault it is that they have not succeeded so far. Rita wants Greg to offer her some real motivation, and blames him for offering her lectures instead. Greg wants to help Rita get moving, and blames her for getting mad when he tries to "tell it like it is" and kick her in the butt. Their positions will not be easy to reconcile, but Greg tries anyway by reminding Rita of their shared goals and his unsuccessful attempts to motivate her in the past.

Greg: I understand that you want to keep the weight down, and so do I.

Rita: I want us to both be skinny, to both be thin.

Greg: But I try to motivate you every morning.

Rita: Motivating me to go to work is different. When have you had to kick me in the butt to go for a walk?

Greg: Nine o'clock at night every night for the last six months.

Rita: You want to go for a walk at nine o'clock at night?

Greg: We could every night. Absolutely!

Rita: So, nine o'clock at night after we've got a Lamaze class and then we've got to visit your grandmother?

Greg: You're making excuses now.

Rita: No. No, Greg, I am not. But we really have been busy.

Greg: I understand that. But every time you've mentioned wanting to go for a walk, whether there's something on TV or not, I'll go for a walk.

Rita: Ummm . . . Frankly, last time it was pretty difficult to get you out to go for a walk. "Oh . . . I don't really want to go." And then finally you said, "Okay, I'll go."

Greg: You're absolutely right, I need to get up off my butt. If you want to walk, I'll definitely get up and walk with you, and that's how I feel. If you have the motivation to get up and walk, anytime you want to walk, I'll walk with you.

Rita: Promise?

Greg: *[joking]* Unless I'm in my underwear on the couch.

Rita: *[not getting it]* See! You can put some tennis shoes on, you can—

Greg: Fine, fine. And I'll make you do that too.

When Greg and Rita speak in generalities, they are in perfect agreement: they both want to lose weight, and they each want the other to be a source of support and motivation. Seems simple, but the devil, alas, lies in the details. Every time they might have actually gone for a walk, there has been a reason not to go, and each one names the other as the one getting in the way. Greg sees himself as extending invitations, and sees Rita as the one making excuses. Rita can recall only times when Greg was the reluctant one, making his promises to accept her invitations ring hollow. Eventually, they manage to move their conversation forward, but sorting out the details of what kind of activity they might pursue together still gets in their way.

Rita: Who has to kick who in the butt when I was doing my exercise videos?

Greg: There's a big difference. Because I don't like exercise tapes! I never liked aerobics. I never had any ambition to do aerobics. Nothing.

Rita: You were doing them for me, you said.

Greg: I was.

Rita: And you promised me you were going to do it.

Greg: It was awful. Awful.

Rita: You only did it once!

Greg: You laughed at me.

Rita: Aw, you were so cute! You were so cute!

Greg: See? It's because you laughed at me.

Rita: I didn't laugh at you Greg, I laughed with you. Because you were laughing too. You're uncoordinated! I told you it gets easier. It was hard for me too.

Aerobics might work for Rita, but it does not work for Greg. Given Rita's previous reaction, it seems unlikely that Greg will voluntarily sign up for another class anytime soon. So the desire to find an activity they can share becomes another obstacle and has the ironic effect of keeping them from doing anything at all. Toward the end of their conversation, the well-worn paths of their struggles over exercise become clear as Greg steers the conversation away from aerobics and back toward taking walks.

Greg: I don't like that you go to try this and try that. It costs a lot of money to take those exercise classes, and if it hasn't been money well spent in the past, I don't think it's going to be money well spent in the future. The best thing is to get out walking.

Rita: Yes, but it's cold out at five o'clock in the morning or whenever you want to go out walking. It's hard.

Greg: We'll figure out something. It doesn't need to start tomorrow, but we need to do something. It's something we have to pace ourselves into.

Rita: Yeah, that's what I'm saying. After the baby comes, I'll be on maternity leave so we can go for walks in the afternoon. I want to get a good jogger to run around with, even when he's a baby, like one month old. He's used to bouncing around, I walk all day.

Greg: Yeah, but you can't take him out if he is the least bit cold. I don't want you to overdo it.

Greg and Rita end their discussion bogged down in a fruitless power struggle, taking turns shooting down each other's ideas. Exercise classes may work for Rita, but Greg dismisses them as too expensive. Walking makes more sense to Greg, but Rita complains that it is too cold when Greg wants to go. This pattern is so entrenched that even when Rita finally expresses some excitement about walking in the afternoons after their baby is born, Greg responds not by embracing her enthusiasm but by warning her not to "overdo it." In the interests of controlling their decision, Greg ends up implying that their problem is the danger of getting too much exercise, instead of too little.

Why do Greg and Rita keep butting heads like this, when they both share the same desire to lose weight and get active? Whenever a couple contemplates a lifestyle change, they face two challenges. They have to decide what changes they want to make—but first they have to decide how they will decide. Greg and Rita never get past that preliminary challenge. Who gets to choose when and how they will get the exercise they both need? How involved should they be in each other's activities? What's the best way for them to motivate each other without getting in each other's way?

Similar issues arose in chapter 4 when we discussed how couples with different food preferences and different attitudes toward weight loss can negotiate changing their diet. There, you learned how appreciating the Principle of Mutual Influence can help couples think about and coordinate their eating habits. The Principle of Mutual Influence plays a similar role in helping couples figure out how to be more active. In this chapter, we will talk about how couples can manage the conflicts that arise when both partners have different approaches to exercise. We will suggest specific ways that partners can exploit their mutual influence to help each other get the exercise that they both need to be healthy and keep fit. But first, we will consider how the challenges of being active are different from the challenges of eating right.

EATING RIGHT AND MOVING MORE:
TWO WAYS TO GET FIT

Research on the health benefits of exercise has been extensive and the results could not be clearer: regular physical activity is crucial for good health. Among older adults, the difference between moving and sitting still can be the difference between life and death. For example, across numerous studies of the effects of exercise on mortality from disease (including research on high blood pressure, diabetes, heart disease, stroke, and cancer), one review calculated that regular exercise decreases mortality by 30 to 35 percent, and extends life expectancy by four to seven years. The benefits are not merely physical. Older adults who get regular exercise report higher quality of life and greater satisfaction than older adults who are sedentary. And it's not just older adults: even healthy young people report feeling significantly better about themselves on days when they have gotten some physical activity. In fact, the ability of exercise to improve emotional well-being is so great that exercise is now being prescribed as a treatment for depression, and in one study it has proven to be as effective as Zoloft (and much cheaper).

When it comes to weight loss, exercise is not quite as effective as eating a better diet, perhaps because it is nearly impossible to exercise hard enough to burn off the calories in one unhealthy meal, let alone a lifetime of them. For example, according to the website Weightloss.com, a 170-pound man would have to jog six miles to burn off the calories in one plain hamburger with a side of fries. To lose weight or keep the weight off, making healthier food choices is a far more efficient strategy, especially in the short term. Yet even if exercise is not a straight path to weight loss by itself, exercise in combination with dietary changes can be the cement that turns short-term weight loss into permanent change. One review of more than 700 studies concluded that, among overweight people, programs focusing on diet plus exercise produced significantly greater reductions in weight, and longer maintenance of weight loss when the program was over, compared with programs focused exclusively on dieting.

So exercise is like a seasoning for life: adding it makes us feel better about ourselves, improves our emotional well-being, promotes physical health and longevity, and, for those who want to lose weight, makes dieting more effective. Given all these benefits, it is poignant that taking full advantage of this cure-all is so difficult for so many of us. Being active takes time and energy, and, in our hyperconnected world, both are in short supply. The recommended activity levels for healthy adults vary depending on who is doing the recommending, but one representative set of guidelines suggests that a healthy adult should get some kind of exercise (brisk walking will do it) for thirty minutes a day, and resistance training (e.g., lifting weights) at least twice a week. In a report from 2010, the Surgeon General of the United States concluded that the majority of Americans are not coming anywhere near to meeting these guidelines. On the contrary, less than half of adults in the United States reach currently recommended levels of physical activity, and 25 percent of all adults report engaging in no physical activity at all on a weekly basis.

As we have seen with healthy eating, there seems to be a large gap between the activity that people need to stay healthy, and the activity that most people are actually getting. When we discussed the problem of eating right in chapter 4, we explained how the Principle of Mutual Influence offers tools for closing that gap. Because our partners are so intimately involved with how, when, and what we eat, it makes sense that partners can be each other's best allies in making difficult dietary changes stick. Are the issues the same with respect to getting more exercise? Can the next three chapters be duplicates of the last three, with the words *moving more* replacing the words *eating right*?

In fact, being more active and eating a healthier diet do raise some similar issues for couples. Both kinds of changes certainly require that couples coordinate and negotiate in ways that sometimes take them by surprise. Indeed, when we were beginning our research for this book, we assumed that the issues would be identical, and that we would be able to talk about diet and exercise at the same time. But when we actually started listening to couples talking about their struggles with diet and their struggles with exercise, we were struck not by the similarities but by the differences. The more couples we heard from, the more convinced we became that getting more exercise raises some issues for couples that they do not face when they talk about eating better.

Specifically, we identified three unique challenges in couples' conversations about being more active:

1. Eating is primarily a social activity, but exercise does not have to be. As we noted in earlier chapters, shared meals anchor our most cherished holidays and celebrations. There are no comparable traditions to support getting regular exercise. Most everyone has Thanksgiving Dinner, but very few families have Thanksgiving Touch Football. Many people have had "business lunches," but very few people have had "business walks." Instead of exercise being woven into our relationships, exercise is often something we engage in outside of our relationships. As a result, couples thinking about eating better have to figure out how to eat better *together*, but couples thinking about getting more exercise have the additional challenge of negotiating how much of that activity they want to do together and how much they are comfortable doing apart.

2. Every one of us has to eat several times a day, but we do not have to exercise. Couples who talk about improving their diets talk about making different choices, but they know they have to choose *something*. Moving more, in contrast, raises the challenge of doing something instead of nothing. It is dangerously easy to avoid exercise altogether, and many people who are not naturally drawn to physical activities do just that. So the difference between eating better and moving more is the difference between resisting things we like and adopting behaviors we may not like. Partners talking about exercise have to find ways to get themselves—and

each other—to do things that, for some people, might be unfamiliar, uncomfortable, or even unpleasant.

3. Our lives are structured around meals, but not around opportunities for physical activity. Every child in school and most workers,
from the office to the construction site, get a lunch hour, whether
they eat lunch during that hour or not. The law does not similarly
protect our time for physical activity. Our days are not naturally
scheduled around exercise unless we schedule it intentionally.
Couples discussing food can take for granted that they will find
the time to eat, but couples discussing exercise have to figure out
when they will find time to move, and what other activities their
time spent exercising is going to displace.

In observing couples talking about exercise, we have seen how easy
it is to get tripped up and bogged down by these challenges. Just like
couples concerned about their diets, couples struggling to get more
exercise return to our research rooms year after year with the same concerns about their lack of physical activity.

The good news is that, although the challenges are new, the basic
principles of relationships that we have been describing throughout this
book continue to apply. In particular, coordinating to get more exercise
requires that couples appreciate the Principle of Mutual Influence and
recognize that working together can overcome these obstacles more effectively than working alone. In the rest of this chapter, we will examine
some of these challenges in more detail:

1. We will describe three characters—the *Outsourcer*, the *Tag-Along*,
and the *Lone Wolf*—that represent extreme answers to the question of how much partners should exercise together versus alone.

2. We will discuss how to support partners who simply have *no taste
for exercise*.

3. We will consider the challenge of *finding time to exercise* in
schedules that are overbooked already.

For each challenge, we will show how smart couples can use their mutual influence to overcome these obstacles and get moving.

WORK OUT TOGETHER OR GO IT ALONE?: THE OUTSOURCER, THE TAG-ALONG, AND THE LONE WOLF

It is easier to get active when others are getting active with us and cheering us on. Exercise books and programs know this, so they usually repeat advice that at first sounds simple: find a workout buddy. Those who can afford it hire personal trainers for exactly this reason, but people in relationships have what could be the perfect personal trainer already at hand. At the crucial moments of decision—when we are choosing whether or not to get out of bed that extra hour before work, or whether to take that walk after dinner instead of falling onto the couch—the ones most likely to be nearby to influence those choices are our partners.

As many of the couples in our studies have discovered, however, involving our partners in exercise is rarely that easy or straightforward. Both members of a couple do not necessarily have the same schedule. Both partners do not always enjoy the same physical activities, or have the same capacity for exercise. And, whereas some types of exercise (like taking a class or playing basketball) double as social activities, other types of exercise (like swimming laps or running on a treadmill) do not. How much should we exercise together and how much should we give each other space to exercise individually? How can we pursue physical fitness as a shared goal and still respect that we may have different approaches to reaching that goal?

In our research, we have seen how couples struggle with the tension between their desire to spend active time together and the recognition that they prefer different ways of being active. Unlike with diets, where couples are going to have to share meals a lot of the time, the issue of exercise allows couples some flexibility to choose how much they are going to exercise together and how much they are going to exercise apart. In navigating this choice, couples can fall into at least three different traps, each of which arises from coming down too hard on one side of this tension or the other.

Consider, for example, the couples who take the idea of a workout buddy very seriously, insisting that the only way they will do any exercise is if both partners can do it together. When both partners are equally committed to physical fitness, this can be a great idea. Exercise programs are indeed more effective and lead to longer-lasting changes in activity levels when partners participate in those programs as a team. But when partners are not equally committed, or prefer different activities, the requirement that both partners always exercise together can be a burden. The message *"I would love it if you would do this activity with me"* can quickly devolve into *"I am not going to do this activity unless you do it with me."* What starts out as a reasonable desire to exercise together becomes an excuse not to exercise.

This is the pattern of the *Outsourcer*, who loads responsibility for exercising onto a reluctant partner so that that person can be blamed when the physical activity does not happen. The husband in the next couple is a perfect example. While in our research rooms, he discussed how much he wants to get back into the shape he was in in college, telling his wife that he would love to go on long, calorie-burning bike rides, if only she would join him. They are a sweet couple, clearly in love, and at first his invitation sounded sweet as well. But as their conversation went on, it soon became clear that they had had this conversation many times before, and she had already told him that bike riding was just not her thing. Wondering why an idea she rejected before keeps coming up, she sensed a hidden agenda at work, and she did not like it.

W: If you say you like to ride the bike, go ride the bike! Why do I
   have to go ride the bike with you?
H: Because, well, I kind of like you to come with me.

W: I know you do! But I don't get anything out of it. Okay, fine, it's nice to do it one day, but it's not like I enjoy it. I don't want to go on these long, twelve-mile rides.

H: We don't have to ride to the lake. We can go on the bike trails.

W: I don't WANT to go on the bike trails! Why don't you understand that?

H: Because it upsets me.

W: Well, I don't understand why. I can like certain things and I don't have to like other things. Why do I have to like what you want me to like?

H: Because, you're my . . .

W: Because I'm your wife.

H: Because you're my wife. You're my buddy!

W: I don't have to be your only buddy, do I?

H: No, but you're my best buddy!

He wants to spend time with his wife, and she wants to support her husband in getting more exercise. So why are they both upset and frustrated? From his perspective, he is feeling rejected by his "best buddy." He cannot imagine that his invitation, coming from the heart, could be read as anything other than affectionate. But it does not come across that way to his wife, for two reasons. First, she also wants to be heard. She has told him clearly, and is telling him again in this conversation, that she is not a fan of bike riding. For him to continue to offer her bike rides only reinforces her suspicion that the invitation is not about her needs at all, but his.

That's frustrating enough, but she has a second reason to be wary: she can sense that he is positioning her as the reason for his reluctance to take any of those bike rides himself. Her being his best buddy has somehow become an excuse for his not exercising alone, and that makes his suggestion of a bike ride together feel like an obligation, rather than an invitation. She tries to break out of this cycle, encouraging him to go ride without her. This Outsourcer will not be denied, however, and he changes the problem from his lack of exercise to her unwillingness to share in an activity he likes. To move toward their goals, he will need to take more responsibility for his own physical activity. But the fact that his behavior is wrapped in genuine affection makes their trap extremely hard to recognize, and harder still to escape.

In some couples, this pattern is reversed: one partner wants to get more exercise, and the other partner gets in the way by insisting that they work out together or not at all. This is the pattern of the *Tag-Along*. Like an anxious younger sibling, the Tag-Along is afraid of being left behind but at the same time makes it much harder to leave the house. Whereas Outsourcers have trouble taking responsibility for their own physical activity, Tag-Alongs won't let their partners take responsibility for their own physical activity, even when doing so would allow both partners to be more active.

The wife in the next couple is an example of a Tag-Along. When we saw them in our research rooms, her husband enthusiastically described several ways that he could get more exercise, including going to the gym, taking walks, and swimming laps in their community pool. His wife supported each choice, but only if she could join him, and there was always some reason why she could not. A few minutes into their conversation, he was getting frustrated.

> **H:** I want to be able to exercise but I like to do it at different times than you do and then you make me feel guilty like, "Why don't you want to do it together?"
>
> **W:** Well, when you were at the gym you were just doing the weight stuff and you need to be doing the cardiovascular stuff.
>
> **H:** But I was! I was walking and stuff like that, but you don't like to do that. I like to do a brisk walk in the morning for an hour, and you like to go strolling around the subdivision for about twenty minutes and then you're like, let's go. And when we go down to the pool, you do five laps and then you're done.

W: Sweetheart, we go walking a lot more than we go to the pool. But if you want to go walking in the mornings, then fine. I've been waking up early, so if you want to try—

H: I think a lot of times it's more feasible to not do it together than together.

W: Then that has to take priority, because I don't feel like I have to lose weight.

H: Okay, as long as that's okay, because you always go, "Oh, well I want to go too. Why can't you wait for me?" And if I want to do something, I want to get an hour done a day, and if you happen to be there then you can come with me or do half the time.

W: Right, but if I'm at home then I don't think you need to shut me out.

A lot of the couples we see discussing exercise are looking for the motivation to get more active. Not this guy. He is clearly eager to hit the gym, or wake up early and walk, or go down to the pool. But each time he tries, he's held back by his partner saying, "Wait for me!" If their desires for exercise matched and their schedules overlapped, this would be a reasonable request. However, as their conversation reveals, she is far less motivated than he is—because, unlike him, she does not feel as though she needs to lose weight. So why does she insist on doing all of their exercise together? She confesses the real issue at the end: she is afraid of being shut out. If they addressed her real concern honestly and directly, the two of them might have found other ways to solve it, but their conversation quickly returned to their difficulties in coordinating schedules. As was true with the Outsourcer, the requirement that they do all their exercise together ended up getting in the way of their fitness more than it helped.

The Outsourcer and the Tag-Along both believe that, in a conflict between the demands of physical fitness and the demands of the relationship, the relationship must win every time. Other partners acknowledge the same conflict but resolve it differently. The *Lone Wolf* is a partner who likes to exercise—a lot—and so demands the right to exercise whenever and however he or she wants. The possibility that these choices may affect the relationship is dismissed as irrelevant because, in the conflict between physical fitness and the relationship, physical fitness must win every time. Whereas the Outsourcer and the Tag-Along are willing to sacrifice their health because the relationship matters too much, the Lone Wolf represents their polar opposite, unwilling to compromise because the relationship does not matter enough.

That is the case for this next couple. The husband is a Lone Wolf, satisfied with the plenty of exercise he gets from his physically demanding job. His wife had been looking for ways to get more active too, and at first she thought her husband might help. By the time they reached our research rooms, however, she suspected that her husband would not be enthusiastic about her request, and she was right.

W: I think it would help me more if you would do something with me. Some type of exercise. I would like it better I think if we could do something together, but I know you hate that.

H: I do hate it. I work all day long.

W: It's just that going by myself kind of sucks.

H: Don't do it because of me, do it for yourself.

W: Well, I *do* do it for myself, but I'm also saying I think it would help me if you would do it with me.

H: I'm not going to, though. I do my exercise at work all day long, all day. I exercise all day long. I don't sit down for ten minutes. That's my exercise. I don't have time to go to the gym and work out. That's just not me. And I'm sure as hell not going to do what you want to do. I'm not going to spin or any of that other garbage.

When partners are talking about losing weight, we hear many say, "*Don't do it for me,*" and usually they mean "*I love you just the way you are.*" For this husband, however, "*Don't do it for me*" means "*Don't involve me in your plans in any way.*" His wife reasonably points out that exercising for herself is perfectly consistent with getting support from him, but he flatly denies her. By the end of his tirade against the gym, this husband's message comes through loud and clear: she is on her own.

The traps that ensnare all three characters stem from the assumption that partners in relationships must choose between doing all of their exercise together (the Outsourcer and the Tag-Along), or none of it together (the Lone Wolf). The narrow range of those choices reflects a misunderstanding of the Principle of Mutual Influence. As we discussed before, mutual influence means that partners in a relationship are always and unavoidably affected by each other's behaviors. When it comes to physical activity, one implication is that everything we do affects our partners' ability to get more exercise. Sharing the same activities is one way, but what the Outsourcer and the Tag-Along miss is that it is not the only way. Partners in a couple can exercise separately and still influence and support each other's fitness goals. In contrast, what the Lone Wolf misses about mutual influence is that the decision not to participate in our partners' efforts to get exercise also affects them. When two people are in a relationship, staying out of each other's business is just not possible.

Are You or Your Partner an Outsourcer, a Tag-Along, or a Lone Wolf?

If you or your partner recognize yourselves in one of these traps, how can you get out? Escaping is as simple as recognizing that you have more options than you think.

RECOGNIZE THAT SOMETIMES THE BEST WAY TO SUPPORT OUR PARTNERS' HEALTH IS TO GRANT THEM SPACE AND TIME ALONE. It is wonderful when two partners want to spend every waking minute together, but even the most adoring couples step away from each other occasionally. Giving our partners space and time to take care of their individual needs is one of the many ways that we care for them. Creating opportunities for our partners to exercise, even if we are not going to be exercising with them, falls into this category of care.

The following husband is a master of this strategy. He is married to an Outsourcer, but instead of getting frustrated by how she unloads responsibility for her exercise on him, he accepts that responsibility in a different way:

H: You need more exercise, so here's what I suggest: I think you should go to the gym after work and spend about an hour working out. We'll get home at the same time, and then after dinner we can take Floyd for a walk. So then Floyd gets walked; you can exercise; I get exercise; and everyone's happy.

W: We've said all this before.

H: Well, not really. I mean if you just say to yourself—make it a rule: you're going to the gym after work.

W: Yes, but the traffic is horrible. It took me thirty minutes to get there the last time I went there straight from work. I didn't get there until 5:40.

H: Maybe you can find other ways to get there. But 5:40 is reasonable because if you leave at 6:40, we'll get home about the same time.

W: *[thinking]* Yeah, but then I—I mean, I don't want to be rushed. I feel like I have to get there exactly when you're going to get there.

H: *[tenderly]* Well, you don't. You can get there after, before, whenever, you know. But you just go to the gym, when you get there you stay for an hour or so, do your workout, and then you leave and come home. You don't have to base it on when I'm going to get home. If I get home first, then I'll start dinner, and that's one less thing for you to worry about.

This husband knows his wife well. He knows that, for her health, she needs to be more physically active. He also knows that she finds excuses not to exercise, and that needing to get home at the same time as he does has been one of those excuses. Some of the partners we have seen might have withdrawn in frustration or responded with criticism ("*Do you want to exercise, or not?!*"). But this husband steps up by removing the obstacles that might have prevented his wife from getting to the gym. He explicitly frees her from the requirement that they arrive home at the same time: "*You can get there after, before, whenever.*" He assures her that he can start dinner without her. Gently but firmly, he refuses to let her undermine her own goals. His example highlights the many ways that we can exploit our connections to our partners to help them exercise, even if we are not always able to exercise with them.

BE WILLING TO TRY NEW THINGS. Everyone likes some kinds of physical activities more than others, and naturally prefers to make time for the ones he or she likes most. In a relationship, however, flexibility is a virtue. The more that both partners are open to exploring new activities, the more they expand the range of activities that they can share together. For couples who want to work out together but have different preferences, finding something active that neither partner has tried before can be a great compromise.

Look how a little openness unlocks the conversation for the following couple. He is the one who wants to return to running, as he used to do regularly when he was younger. She is a Tag-Along: she likes the idea of getting fit together but has never been much of a runner. After he expresses a clear intention to start exercising before work every day, she is faced with a choice, and she makes it.

> **W:** You're going to get up at 5:30 in the morning and go running?
> **H:** That's what I used to do! I used to get up and do that and I lost weight, so I don't mind doing that.
> **W:** Okay. I mean, I'll try too. I'm not a morning person, but I'll try it for . . . I'll give you—
> **H:** I'm not asking you to do it if you don't—
> **W:** No, it would be healthy for me too. Because I enjoy spending

time with you and I think that's something that we have in
common, and I'd rather do that together than do that separately.
But I also love to go on bike rides with you, and it would be great
if we could get back in the habit of doing that too.

What could have been a conflict evaporates with "*I'll try.*" Those
words send two messages. First, she indicates that her desire to get fit
together is sincere. He is offering her a way of supporting him in getting more exercise, and she is taking it. Second, she indicates that, for his
sake and for the sake of their health, she is willing to do things that do
not come naturally to her. That's a powerful way to care for someone
you love. Her openness has another advantage too—he's more likely to
reciprocate when she suggests they ride bikes together.

DO IT ALL! EXERCISE ALONE AND TOGETHER. Sometimes we have to choose
one path over another, but not always. One reason that Lone Wolves
may react badly to an invitation to work out together is that they perceive it as a threat to effective workout schedules they have already
established. This is an experience worth validating, because setting
up—and following!—an exercise schedule is a real accomplishment.
If your partner is a Lone Wolf, consider defusing this threat by directly
acknowledging the value of his or her existing routines and respecting
them. In this way, working out together can be an additional way of
getting exercise, rather than a sacrifice.

FOR PARTNERS WHO HATE TO EXERCISE:
THE MIRACLE OF REWARD SUBSTITUTION

For people unaccustomed to physical activity, the prospect of getting
regular exercise can be daunting. Gymnasiums can be scary to the un-
initiated, full of unfamiliar people working on intimidating machines.
The expression *No pain, no gain* suggests that, in order to benefit us,

exercise has to hurt. That does not sound too attractive. It is not surprising that many people consider their options and just say no.

If you are concerned about your partner's health and discussing the possibility of getting more exercise, a gut-level distaste for getting sweaty is a hard obstacle to overcome. Indeed, among the couples who visit our research rooms to talk about getting more exercise, this is where we have seen many conversations crash into a wall. The next couple is a good example. Recognizing that their sedentary lifestyle is putting them at risk, the husband is gung ho to add regular exercise to their lives. The wife does not dispute the fact that more physical activity would be good for them, but that is not enough to get her moving.

> **H:** Okay, we're talking about exercise. I just think we should do more
> active things, like locally, like on Saturday or Sunday. We could go
> for a bike ride, or walk the dog. We can do that every night; we
> could walk her for a half hour around the block. That's good for
> us and good for her. We just need something more—something
> that is more of an activity.
>
> **W:** *[skeptically]* I'm not an activity type of person. Everybody
> knows that you're supposed to get exercise. I just don't like
> doing it.
>
> **H:** Well, that's why we need to do stuff that makes it more of an
> activity, not just exercise. I mean, I kind of like going and running
> on the treadmill and watching a TV show or whatever, but I know
> you don't like that. But you don't mind bike riding, do you? You
> might like it if we find a nice place to ride. And there are lots of
> trails around here that are real good.
>
> **W:** But I'm scared of having a bicycle I need a degree to operate.
>
> **H:** *[puzzled]* What do you mean?
>
> **W:** I've never ridden a bike with gears.
>
> **H:** *[slowly]* Well, the gears are usually—
>
> **W:** And my feet don't touch the ground.

H: Well, if your feet did touch the ground, you couldn't really pedal very well. Because you know when your pedal is to the bottom, your leg has to be pretty straight.

W: Yeah, but I have very short legs.

You have to give this husband credit for persistence. Every time he makes a suggestion, his wife has a reason why it won't work, but he keeps right on trying. Nevertheless, it was clear that this conversation was going nowhere from the moment she declared, "*I just don't like doing it.*" No amount of arguing is going to change her mind, any more than someone who hates vegetables, French films, or abstract paintings can be persuaded to appreciate them.

The husband in the next example takes the same stand against exercise, but his wife responds in a different way. Whereas the previous husband kept on making suggestions, only to see each one knocked down, the wife in this next couple directs the spotlight squarely on her husband's reluctance. This turns out to be a strategy that opens some doors.

H: I don't like to exercise.

W: Okay.

H: So what are we going to do, then?

W: I'm not going to do anything. What are you going to do?

H: I need to decide, for myself. Actually, the decision is there. I want to do something about it.

W: Then why haven't you?

H: Because I'm a lazy ass.

W: I see.

H: And when I get pushed, I push back.

W: Have you decided to change your mind about being a lazy ass? Or is that still kind of up in the air?

H: That's still kind of up in the air, I guess.

W: Okay. Well, let me know when you decide to change your mind.

Notice how effective a few simple questions can be. This wife could have jumped in with suggestions like the husband in the previous example, but she chooses not to. Instead, her reasonable questions place the responsibility for initiating a change onto her husband where it belongs. Whereas the wife in the previous example could blame her failure to exercise on her husband's inadequate suggestions, the husband in this couple has no one to blame. As a result, his bold assertion that *"the decision is there"* deflates rather quickly to the admission that, in fact, his decision is *"still kind of up in the air."* This husband, in recognizing his own role in his lack of physical activity, is several steps ahead of the prior wife, even if he still has no concrete ways to get past the fact that he just does not like to exercise.

Do You or Your Partner Just Hate to Exercise?

So what can you do? The trick is to get past the dread and transform exercise into something enjoyable, or, failing that, into something bearable that you do for the sake of good health. This is of course the explicit reason why people purchase gym memberships or sign up for aerobics classes: exercising around other people offers the chance to turn what might otherwise be a chore into a social event. The reason that so many gym memberships go unused, however, is that it is hard to develop powerful relationships with people we meet and interact with infrequently. For someone who does not like to work out, seeing that casual acquaintance on the next StairMaster is not a particularly strong motivator.

On the other hand, our intimate relationships can be sources of motivation for us. In fact, as the Principle of Mutual Influence points out, our partners are unique in their power to transform ordinary, or even unpleasant, activities into events we can look forward to. Partners who take advantage of their mutual influence over each other have two effective ways to get each other moving more, even when exercising is the last thing either partner wants to do:

RESIST NARROW DEFINITIONS OF EXERCISE. One reason that some people insist that they do not like working out is that they define exercise exclusively as "something people do with heavy, expensive machinery at a gym." But exercise has been around a lot longer than the Stair-Master. Compared with sitting on the couch, *any* physical activity offers significant health benefits. You can be the one to remind your reluctant partner of that fact, and encourage a more open, creative approach to being active.

So maybe your partner does not enjoy running, but how about walking or hiking? Your partner may not be an athlete, but he or she might still be tempted by salsa dancing or ice skating. Even window-shopping down a commercial street is more active than shopping online. The point is that we all have something we like to do that will get us off the couch. You can use your influence to help your partner find that new and exciting activity. If you make it a date night, then it's not exercise.

PRACTICE REWARD SUBSTITUTION. Some chores never become fun, but we faithfully do them anyway because they get us closer to something we want that we cannot get any other way. We want healthy teeth and gums, so we brush our teeth and floss. We care about our appearance, so we do laundry and fold our clothes. The link between the chore and the reward is what keeps us doing the chore. Behavioral economist Dan Ariely has suggested that, whenever we are confronted with a task that we do not inherently enjoy but know we have to do, we should purposefully pair that activity with something that we do enjoy. This is called *reward substitution*.

In a good relationship, being together can be the reward that makes exercise something to look forward to. You might get bored running on the treadmill, but if your partner meets you at the gym after work, the chore becomes a cherished hour to catch up on the events of the day. Even if you and your partner cannot arrange your schedules to exercise together, you can use your knowledge of each other's preferences to set up reward substitutions. Sure, your partner may normally hate that stationary bike gathering dust in the corner of the bedroom, but if you both agree that you can play back the latest episodes of *Top Chef* from your DVR only when you are riding it, then the time spent exercising becomes a means to a desirable end.

FOR THE PERSON WITH NO TIME: ECONOMIES OF SCALE IN RELATIONSHIPS

"Exercise? I'd love to, but who has the time?" Do you know anyone who is looking for *more* things to do? A too-full schedule is the chronic problem of modern life, and one of the major reasons people cite to explain why they are not more physically active. Moreover, it is a reasonable excuse. Yes, exercise is important, but so are all the other things that keep us busy throughout the day.

Perhaps you can empathize with the following wife, a former nursing student now running her husband's medical practice, who explained her situation while visiting our research rooms.

> There's no time. When I worked at the VA, I'd come home and
> I was always so tired there was nothing I could do. But at least
> when I was at the VA I was walking. I walked up and down stairs, I
> walked across the hospital, I always walked at least fifteen minutes
> to thirty minutes every day. Regardless if I wanted to do it or not,
> I always had some form of exercise. Now at the office, I'm sitting
> there answering the phones, and that's about it. So I don't do as
> much as I'd like to, and I guess that's my biggest problem. I can't
> find the time.

Who hasn't had this complaint recently? When the work is piling up and the walls are closing in, putting off exercise until tomorrow, next week, or next month, makes a lot of sense. The problem is that, for most of us, life is not going to get any less busy anytime soon. Those who are postponing exercise "until things calm down" are likely to be waiting a long time, and getting no healthier while they wait.

If You and Your Partner Can't Find Time to Exercise

When our responsibilities are piling up and the number of hours in a day refuses to extend beyond the usual twenty-four, the Principle of Mutual Influence offers a way out. The fact is that couples working together toward a shared goal can, if they try, be far more efficient than partners working alone. The economist Adam Smith referred to this as *economies of scale,* a term he used to describe the fact that larger organizations can frequently produce goods more cost-effectively than smaller ones. Economies of scale explain why the health insurance purchased through a large employer usually costs less than health insurance purchased by individuals, and why Walmart, the largest retailer on the planet, can sell products more cheaply than any other store. At first, a couple may not seem like a "larger organization" compared with a single person, but consider that a group of two is 100 percent larger than a group of one. Doubling the number of people available to maintain a home opens a lot of doors to increased efficiency. Couples who recognize and exploit this fact have a number of ways to carve out time for exercise in even the busiest overscheduled lives.

DIVIDE AND CONQUER. A lot of the efficiencies of larger organizations come from the skillful division of labor. When a task is complex, different people taking on different aspects of the task can do so more effectively than one person trying to do everything. Maintaining a household is certainly complex, and so the same principle applies. For example, both partners do not have to go grocery shopping; if one partner shops, that frees the other to help children with homework, or pay bills, or take care of some other errand that needs doing. A couple who cannot find the time to exercise together can still take care of each partner's health by taking care of each other's chores, buying time for each other to get some kind of exercise on a regular basis. Some partners make explicit bargains with each other: I'll go to the gym at night while you bathe the kids and get them ready for bed, and you can go to the gym in the morning while I am feeding them breakfast and getting them ready for school. A secondary advantage of this sort of bargain is that knowing our partners are picking up the slack for us while we work out may drive us to work out that much harder.

MAKE IT A HABIT. People who have lost weight and kept it off describe how eating right and exercising regularly became habits that they eventually stopped planning and just did, like getting out of bed in the morning. We don't have to develop the habit of eating—even if we had no memory for mealtimes, our hunger would remind us. But, if we are not accustomed to it, we do have to develop the habit of exercising regularly. Once exercising regularly becomes ingrained, we do not have to make time for it, because we will have already done so. It's the other tasks of life that we will have to make time for. One husband in our research rooms expressed this idea perfectly:

> I think that it's important to keep it [exercise] part of our routine so
> that it's just something that we do, and it'll feel sort of awkward if we
> *don't* do it.

But how to create a new habit of an activity that is all too easy to postpone, forget, or avoid? By assuming that you are going to exercise no matter what. After dinner, initiate a walk around the neighborhood instead of collapsing onto the couch. That precious weekend morning is no less precious if it becomes an active morning for both of you. Sure, it would be great if you and your partner could take turns getting you both moving, but if your partner is the more reluctant one, better that you take the lead than both of you miss getting some activity. You can be the cue that reminds your partner when it's time to get active, like a living (and loving) human Post-it note.

KEY POINTS FROM CHAPTER 7

- Many of the challenges of moving more are similar to the challenges of eating right, but getting more active also raises unique issues.

- One challenge for couples is deciding how much to exercise together and how much to exercise alone. When partners come down too hard on either side of this choice, they tend to fall into recognizable traps. Some partners (the *Outsourcer* and the *Tag-Along*) insist on always working out together, and in so doing make it almost impossible to get any exercise at all, effectively making each other responsible for their own reluctance to get moving. Other partners (the *Lone Wolf*) refuse to compromise their own exercise routines. Their persistence and dedication can be inspiring, but they are missing opportunities to help mates who have not yet developed such routines. The way out of these traps is to be flexible: realize that making an effort to exercise together *and* giving a partner space to exercise alone are both ways to show how much we care about our partners' health.

- Some people simply dislike physical activity, and for these partners we can practice reward substitution, pairing exercise they may not enjoy with valued rewards, like time together or a chance to see a favorite film or television show.

- Partners who have difficulty finding time to exercise can take advantage of economies of scale, taking on each other's tasks to buy time for each other to exercise when there is not enough time to exercise together.

PLANNING FOR CHANGE

Each of the statements below describes something that successful couples do to sustain each partner's efforts to stay active. For each one, consider how well you and your partner engage in this behavior, and how easy or difficult it will be for the two of you to make any needed improvements.

1. We *respect* each other's different preferences when it comes to exercise.
   ____ This is a real strength for us. We do not need to make changes in this area.
   ____ We could improve in this area, and we think it will be easy to do so.
   ____ We could improve in this area, but we think it will be difficult to do so.

2. We *strike a balance* between sharing physical activities together and granting each other space to exercise alone.
   ____ This is a real strength for us. We do not need to make changes in this area.
   ____ We could improve in this area, and we think it will be easy to do so.
   ____ We could improve in this area, but we think it will be difficult to do so.

3. We are *flexible and open* to trying new kinds of physical activities.
   ____ This is a real strength for us. We do not need to make changes in this area.
   ____ We could improve in this area, and we think it will be easy to do so.
   ____ We could improve in this area, but we think it will be difficult to do so.

4. We *practice reward substitution,* linking exercise with rewards that both of us want.
   ____ This is a real strength for us. We do not need to make changes in this area.
   ____ We could improve in this area, and we think it will be easy to do so.
   ____ We could improve in this area, but we think it will be difficult to do so.

5. We are willing to *take on each other's household tasks* to buy each other time for regular exercise.
   ____ This is a real strength for us. We do not need to make changes in this area.

____ We could improve in this area, and we think it will be easy to do so.

____ We could improve in this area, but we think it will be difficult to do so.

If you found yourself marking the first answer a lot, then you and your partner clearly appreciate the Principle of Mutual Influence and have been exploiting that understanding to reinforce each other's efforts to get enough exercise.

If your responses tend toward the second answer, then you know what you need to do. Now that you understand how the Principle of Mutual Influence works, you and your partner have a number of great ways to keep each other on track, and there is nothing stopping you from working together to make exercise a permanent part of your lives.

If you found yourself often marking the third answer, then you and your partner may understand the Principle of Mutual Influence but still recognize that making that influence work for you in your own lives will not be easy. Consider reviewing this chapter again with an eye toward identifying concrete steps that you can take today, remembering that real, measurable benefits come from even small amounts of exercise.

8

Moving More and
Mutual Understanding

LISTENING FOR A CHANGE

WHEN WE FIRST INTERVIEWED Darryl, he was in his early thirties, working as an English and drama teacher.

I was always a pudgy kid, but I got really big after my parents separated. So I was pretty much the depressed fat kid until my junior year in high school, and then I ran track and cross-country and lost it all. College, same deal. I was lean and mean, exercising all the time, feeling great. But now—seriously? No exercise, and I feel like crap, moody, tired all the time. I'm the fat kid again, right back where I started. Used to be large and in charge, now: just large.

Now more than twenty pounds beyond his preferred weight, Darryl had serious doubts about whether he could pull off the same feat again. Equally unhappy with her weight, Darryl's wife, Camilla, a mortgage broker, recounted how active they had been together earlier in their relationship. But then, like many young couples, Darryl and Camilla soon settled into a comfortable routine, working long hours to save money for a down payment on a home. Their exercise habits fell by the wayside, except for occasional bursts of activity, and both added a few pounds with each passing year. Eventually Darryl and Camilla could no longer deny that switching to a healthier lifestyle was necessary and overdue. They were starting to get their eating and snacking habits back under control, but both still felt overweight and wanted to get, in Camilla's words, "lighter and tighter."

When we asked Darryl and Camilla to discuss something that Darryl wanted to change about himself—an issue that could not be a problem in the marriage—he immediately chose "exercising more" as his topic. We left them alone to have a private conversation, and after they exchanged pleasant smiles, the tone of their conversation started to shift.

Darryl: Help me.

Camilla: Well, what do you want to change about yourself?

Darryl: I want to feel better, have more energy, lose weight . . . And so we can look better and so I won't be so *rotund*. I just feel . . . ugh *[grunting]*.

Camilla: You're not *rotund*. I still find you very attractive.

Darryl: Then why do you always call me dough boy?

Camilla: I've never called you dough boy. Bigfoot maybe, but never dough boy.

Darryl: You do it a lot. You called me Pillsbury Dough Boy the other day when I got out of the shower.

Camilla: I still find you attractive. You know that, right?

Darryl: Yeah, whatever.

Let's take a closer look at what Darryl and Camilla are saying to each other here. Overweight and discouraged, Darryl wants to take control of his health and return to a serious exercise regimen. Sounding a bit desperate, he asks Camilla for help but finds little sincerity in her attempts to reassure him that he remains attractive to her. How *could* he be convinced, knowing that her supposedly positive impression of his appearance directly contradicts his own feelings—"*ugh!*"—and her recent teasing?

Next we will see that Darryl's desire to get moving has triggered Camilla's resentment, probably because she feels her opinion on this subject is not so important to him.

> **Camilla:** So you don't want to change because it matters to our relationship? You don't want to change for me?
>
> **Darryl:** No, I want to change for *me*.
>
> **Camilla:** What if I didn't find you attractive anymore and I was embarrassed to be seen with you? Wouldn't you be upset?
>
> **Darryl:** *[surprised, sarcastic]* Well, thanks. I don't know. Probably. What's this have to do with anything?

For reasons Darryl cannot quite fathom, he has struck a nerve in Camilla. He is baffled by the 180-degree turn in her attitude—attracted to him one moment and repulsed the next. When they tacitly agree to drop Camilla's uncomfortable line of questioning, their discussion turns toward the logistics of Darryl's exercise routine. But this is not a problem that can be solved by careful scheduling, because deeper currents of emotion remain unresolved.

> **Camilla:** How do you plan to exercise more? I wanted to do it together. You didn't want to.
>
> **Darryl:** I want to go to a gym.
>
> **Camilla:** Why do we have to go to a gym?
>
> **Darryl:** Because I like it there.
>
> **Camilla:** Well then, I guess you'll have to go to the gym. Go away and spend less time with me.
>
> **Darryl:** Well, I want you to go with me.
>
> **Camilla:** Why do you want me to go with you?

Darryl: So we can spend time together and I can lose weight and exercise.

Camilla: But you won't do stuff with me.

Darryl: You wanted me to get up at 5:30 in the morning and do it with you!

From Darryl's perspective, this is not a complex problem. He is back to being overweight, feels terrible about it, and knows that getting on his feet is a tried-and-true solution. He wants some help and encouragement from Camilla, and if he can go to the gym with her, so much the better—they'd be able to spend time together, after all. But at every turn Darryl meets resistance. As the conversation winds down, Darryl discloses the depths of his fear, only to encounter his greatest obstacle yet.

Camilla: I still don't understand why you think it's a problem.

Darryl: It's a health problem.

Camilla: So you think you're going to die sooner if you don't lose weight?

Darryl: Uh-huh. Have a heart attack.

Camilla: You really think that?

Darryl: Yeah. I just want to look and feel like I did in high school—young and healthy . . . How do you feel about me exercising more, losing weight? Don't you want me to?

Camilla: I'd rather you didn't.

Beneath Camilla's harsh words there seems to be ambivalence over her role as a partner. Camilla wants to be the person Darryl goes to for support and, more important, for approval. She needs to know that Darryl cares about looking good *for her*. If Darryl doesn't acknowledge the importance of Camilla's opinion about him, she's not sure how to back his exercise plan. Camilla feels neglected and can't see a place for her in Darryl's efforts to change. In fact, although she may not recognize it, Camilla's last statement suggests she is threatened by the prospect of Darryl changing.

From Camilla's perspective, Darryl's plan to lose weight means that she'll need to make some drastic changes as well—and she's not ready to sacrifice anything. Unless Darryl agrees to exercise according to her convenience, on her terms, she seems unwilling to help him. Camilla's support comes with strings attached; she requires Darryl to conform to her ideas of when, where, and how to work out. And if he doesn't conform, she'd rather he not lose weight at all.

In our interviews with couples, we often see that when one partner takes the initiative to become healthier, it forces the other partner to confront his or her own weight issues and exercise habits—issues and habits that he or she might rather downplay or flat-out deny. Beyond Camilla's simply feeling neglected, a big part of her unwillingness to help may come from her not being ready to face up to feelings she may have about her own weight. Darryl does not see that he may be putting Camilla into a difficult spot, and Camilla doesn't yet understand that her husband's request for help is churning up important feelings for her— feelings she needs to acknowledge if she is going to be an effective collaborator. Neither partner is clearly right or wrong, but both are stuck just the same, and just a little bit of insight would go a long way toward breaking the logjam that they now face.

Can Darryl and Camilla turn this around? In our laboratory two years later, Darryl—now thirty pounds overweight by his report— echoed his earlier wishes to exercise more and lose weight. Parents of twin girls now, Darryl and Camilla seemed happy to have some quiet time in our lab to catch up. But once again their conversation did not go well. Darryl began by complaining about Camilla's teasing, and she in turn criticized him for always making excuses for not getting to the gym. They also discussed other ways Darryl might exercise, along with Camilla's poor eating habits and the recent news that Camilla's doctor is worried about *her* weight. Darryl and Camilla do not understand each other's health needs very well, and as a result they are ineffective at connecting with and supporting each other.

Darryl and Camilla are not unique. Circumstances and details change from couple to couple, of course, but even this brief excerpt illustrates the basic pattern we see in our studies: One partner, frustrated and maybe even embarrassed, realizes that the time has finally come to get serious about burning calories. Like Darryl, many such partners are worried that their health will worsen if they remain overweight and sedentary, yet they find exercise inconvenient, agonizing, or just plain boring. They would avoid the issue if they could, but they sense—correctly—that the need to exercise will become more urgent and more difficult as time passes. Help-seekers like Darryl want to be reassured and will often disparage themselves (*"I'm rotund!"*) to elicit sympathy. They want to know they can rely on their partners for strength and confidence as they contemplate healthier habits. Genuine support and reasoned guidance are therefore crucial for helping this person become more active. Facing a pretty tall order, the mate tries to help with a variety of strategies, but all too often ends up faltering in four distinct ways: 1) reassuring the partner that everything will be fine, with or without the weight loss; 2) covertly blaming the partner for prior failures; 3) alarming the partner about how dire the situation really is; or 4) limiting the partner's exercise options in some way. Some mates do get it right, but many more seem threatened or bothered by the partner's newfound inspiration and, like Camilla, do little to meet the partner's need for effective support.

TEAMING UP TO MOVE MORE: MIND THE GAP

Though couples like Darryl and Camilla may not realize it, they do have good options for breaking this stalemate. By viewing their problems from the vantage point of our second principle, the Principle of Mutual Understanding, couples can discover a few simple options that bolster rather than block a partner's desire to get more exercise. Mutual understanding is in short supply when Darryl and Camilla discuss their health—that much is obvious. But why do they keep falling into this trap?

In this chapter you will learn how one person's resistance to the partner's desire to exercise—like Camilla's limp support and her tendency to sabotage Darryl's goals—can reflect feelings of threat and inadequacy. And you will learn how one partner's lack of motivation and willingness to forgo exercise—evidenced by Darryl's gradual slide toward inactivity and his pleas for help from Camilla—can reflect self-doubt and uncertainty about the other partner's emotional availability. Our work shows that Camilla's resistance and Darryl's inactivity are paradoxically *rewarded* in situations like this because they inadvertently solve hidden problems for couples. For example, by resisting Darryl's desire to exercise more, Camilla is able to protect herself from feeling threatened and weak. Darryl, on the other hand, is able to confirm that he remains attractive to Camilla, even though his health and appearance are declining. These are the dynamics that couples like Darryl and Camilla are failing to appreciate and, we believe, add to their struggle to be more active.

The Principle of Mutual Understanding is familiar to you from earlier in the book; in chapter 5, we addressed this same principle specifically in relation to eating right. You may recall how the Charmer ("*But you look fantastic!*"), the One-Trick Pony ("*Just do what I did!*"), and the Waffler ("*It's impossible for you to help me, but that won't stop me from asking!*") all generate unique misunderstandings that derail efforts to adopt healthier diets. These ideas also apply to couples' efforts to exercise more—you may have already noticed Camilla's tendency to be a Charmer, for example—but discussions about exercise raise two additional issues that put pressure on partners' understanding of each other.

First, when people talk about exercising more, they often comment specifically on wanting to look better, be more muscular, wear nicer clothes, appear energized and more successful, and tighten up specific parts of their bodies—in short, wanting to do all the things they did to attract their current mates in the first place! Little wonder, then, that *one partner's desire to exercise more might lead the mate to feel insecure and defensive.*

Second, more so than in discussions about eating right, *talking about moving more naturally raises concerns about whether both partners have the same skill levels and preferences for exercise.* Questions arise over who will make accommodations for whom, whether they will be able to exercise in the same place at the same time and, if not, what it means to be partners who value spending a lot of their free time together but choose not to when it comes to working out. As a result, the new emphasis one partner places on his or her physical appearance and personal preferences can come off as selfish and can easily lead to feelings of jealousy, abandonment, and anger.

These kinds of insecurities can lead to two types of destructive patterns that undermine couples' efforts to move more:

1. The *Saboteur,* who comes up with any excuse to derail a partner's exercise regimen, and

2. The *Reassurance Trap,* when one partner constantly reassures the other that he or she looks fine just as is, and doesn't need to exercise . . . even if it's not true.

By revisiting and expanding the Principle of Mutual Understanding, and applying it to this topic of exercise, we'll figure out ways to overcome these common challenges.

SELF-PROTECTION OR AUTHENTIC CONNECTION? THE SABOTEUR

"Are you sure you want to join that gym? It is a bit out of the way, and after the baby comes I worry that the location will be very inconvenient for you."

"I would rather you not go running at night—it is dark, and our neighborhood is not so safe. How about if we walk together in the mornings?"

"I'm no expert, but it sure seems to me that you need to ease yourself into this. Remember what the doctor said about hurting your back and doing things gradually?"

When deciding on new ways to burn more calories, relationship partners brainstorm their way toward what they hope will be smart, sustainable solutions. But do the above statements offer the scaffolding that partners need to make good decisions, or are they roadblocks that will stop them in their tracks? The difference lies beneath the surface of the statements themselves, in whether the speaker genuinely intends to connect with the partner's plans or to protect his or her own immediate self-interests. A first step in applying the Principle of Mutual Understanding here is for both partners to recognize that self-protective statements are covering up the Saboteur's uncertainties and feelings of vulnerability—feelings that the help-seeker is helping to create. Although self-protective statements typically do create resistance and friction for the partner trying to move more, they are not malicious. The problem is not that the Saboteur wants an inactive and lethargic partner; the problem is that the Saboteur wants something else even more: less threat, less anxiety, and less vulnerability.

The following statements, for example, paraphrase the kinds of responses we hear from people after being asked to support their partner's desire to exercise:

- *If you go to the gym, I will be left alone.*
- *If you slim down, I will look worse by comparison.*
- *If you want to exercise more, I will struggle to keep up; I'm just not ready yet.*
- *If you are going to make a decision like this all by yourself, I will feel hurt.*

- *If you are the one getting all the attention, I will feel ignored.*
- *If you hurt yourself again, I'm the one who will have to take care of you.*
- *If you become more attractive to other people, I will feel jealous.*

The underlying sense of discomfort—and even threat—virtually writes the rest of the script to close the internal emotional gaps: *You already look pretty good the way you are! Do you really want to go to the gym? Of course I will go with you, but why do you have to do it at such odd hours?*

However the statement is made, the simple point is that when one partner indicates a readiness to move more and look better, it can initiate a cascade of conflicting reactions in the mate. A perceived threat or a twinge of anxiety triggers the impulse to reduce that discomfort by *resisting* any kind of change, and often leads to efforts to undermine the partner's desire to exercise. Protection of the status quo is preferred over connection with the partner's goals, and promising opportunities for support are missed as a consequence. As tempting as it is for us to dismiss the help-seeker's inactivity as reflecting a simple lack of motivation, and as tempting as it is to label the mate's flaccid support as merely a lack of affection, our work indicates that many couples are negotiating some version of the protection-connection dilemma when they are talking about exercise. And when the helper chooses self-protection over authentic connection, sabotage often follows.

Applying the Principle of Mutual Understanding can go far in helping couples to sidestep these challenges. Consider the following excerpt, in which a woman, Lisa, has asked her husband, Chad, if he would be willing to help her get into better shape. Lisa asked Chad a series of questions about whether he would exercise with her, allow her to purchase a gym membership, and massage her lower back after workouts. Each time Chad's response was sympathetic but curt—"Yeah," "Sure," "Fine, no problem"—but Lisa eventually caught on to the fact that something was wrong:

W: You look like you're pissed. Is this a sore topic?

H: You getting in shape? We already discussed it and we both agree. I've already gone with you to help you do it.

W: Oh yeah.

H: *[mocking, angry]* "Oh yeah." My stepdad has helped, the whole family is behind you, even the kids. Because when *you* want something, we help you along with it.

W: But when you want to do something? I guess I'm not supportive?

H: Why would you say that?

W: Because I guess I'm not supportive of you?

H: I didn't say that, Lisa. What makes you think you're not supportive of me?

W: Would you please stop playing these stupid mind games and tell me what you're mad at?

Just like Darryl, Lisa wants to exercise more, turns to her partner for help, and is surprised by Chad's resistance and hostility. Chad shows little inclination to connect with Lisa's new exercise agenda, opting instead to protect himself and offering only the illusion of support. This is the Saboteur's trademark, and as a result the difficulties that Lisa has faced in trying to exercise on a regular basis are unlikely to go away. We can see that Lisa has put Chad in a difficult position; he is not a Saboteur by choice, he just wants to be appreciated for the support he has already provided.

How might this have gone differently? Clearly Lisa recognizes that her request does not sit well with Chad, and she needs to find out why. To her credit Lisa says, *"I guess I'm not supportive?"* twice, but Chad is having none of it. He does not want to be the one to tell Lisa that she is not supportive of him; he wants her to figure this out on her own, and he wants her to feel bad just like he does. With a deeper appreciation for the feelings at work here, Lisa might have said something like, *"Sorry. I guess my enthusiasm got the better of me. You're right. I've been a bit selfish about this. But now that you point it out, I can see how much your support has*

already mattered to me." She could make it easier for her partner to connect with her rather than protect himself. Real support for Lisa's new
exercise habits will not be forthcoming until she acknowledges Chad's
feelings. By being validated by Lisa, Chad will feel less imposed upon
and more like an equal partner in the relationship, and he will be inclined to give his support more freely.

With greater sensitivity to the emotions and threats stirred up by
discussions about exercise and weight loss, some partners are able to
negotiate a deeper understanding of their respective positions. Consider another example, in which the man is only too aware of his need
to tighten up his physique. A civil rights attorney at a respected firm,
he is increasingly troubled by being sedentary and overweight—in
part because he thinks wearing baggy suits makes him feel less confident on the job. Will his wife feel threatened by his new plan to lose
weight? Married later in life than many of our other couples—both
are in their mid-forties—his wife has managed to stay trim and fit
while he has gained sixty-five pounds over the six years they have
known each other.

> **W:** How do you feel about me and how I see you? Do you think my
> perspective of you has changed as far as the issues we're talking
> about?
>
> **H:** Well, how are you going to feel when I lose all the weight? Is it
> going to be an issue for you with jealousy or—
>
> **W:** What do you mean?
>
> **H:** Are you going to be like, "Gee, he lost all this weight and now he
> feels good about himself and he's going out in public and women
> are going to be flirting with him"?
>
> **W:** We can talk about that later.
>
> **H:** No, but I want to know. It affects me.
>
> **W:** I'll be honest here and say when I think about you as the
> person that you are trying to become physically, of course your
> confidence is going to come back. But then I think, "What if he's

too confident? What if he can't handle being married and getting
that type of attention because he's never been in that situation
before?"

H: I understand what you are saying.

W: Right. We're married now. There are certain things that you
can't do anymore, but you have yet to experience those scenarios
[where you are thin, confident, and married].

H: We should just—I think, we'll see when it happens.

This issue is far from being resolved. The wife may be *over*estimating
how confident her husband will become after he begins to exercise regularly; she also assumes that his confidence will lead to flirtation. He, on
the other hand, may be *under*estimating how threatened and jealous she
feels by the prospect of his losing weight. The way he addresses these
feelings will determine whether she continues to focus on protecting
herself and sabotaging his desire to exercise more, or starts to connect
with him and his desire to be fit and healthy. But this couple is aware of
how his anticipated weight loss could affect them both and they appear
willing to engage difficult issues like this.

As you may have already inferred from this couple, the fact that the
wife is reasonably secure in her own physique probably allows her to
be less threatened by her husband's desire to tone his up. Indeed, this
woman may welcome her husband's shift to a more advanced stage of
change, and even take some private satisfaction in knowing that she
coaxed him toward this healthy decision. And we can imagine that she
would be more defensive and less generous with her support if she were
overweight but unwilling to do much about it. When partners are at
different stages of change, the opportunities for misunderstanding and
the feelings of being threatened can be especially great.

You may recall that Darryl, for example, seemed to be way ahead of
Camilla in wanting to exercise more. And because both partners failed
to see this, Camilla ended up functioning like a brake or an anchor
on the changes Darryl wanted to make. The feeling of threat can be

particularly strong for people in Camilla's position, and so she naturally dug in her heels more than she otherwise would have if she had been closer to Darryl's stage in being ready to exercise.

The husband in the following couple is in pretty good shape but he has let his bike-riding regimen slide. With some free time on his hands now, he is eager to get moving again. His wife, in contrast, has been told by her doctor that she is obese, yet she shows little inclination to exercise more as a way to manage her weight. They are obviously at very different stages of change. They can either succumb to this through resistance and defensiveness, or they can connect through mutual understanding.

> **H:** I really want to start to ride again, start to be fit again, and doing exercises. I need that time every day, so that might be like an hour or two that you're by yourself.
>
> **W:** Sure, if that's what you want to do, we can make that happen.
>
> **H:** And I was also thinking about doing either like a 100-kilometer or 100-mile race.
>
> **W:** Whoa whoa whoa whoa whoa!
>
> **H:** *[openmouthed, shocked]* What? What do you mean?
>
> **W:** Let's not jump ahead of ourselves here! I'm just saying, let's get you back in the routine and then we'll cross that bridge when we get there. . . . But okay, what else?
>
> **H:** Umm, let's see. I want to do Pilates . . .
>
> **W:** Pilates!? We don't live in California. And even if we did, that stuff doesn't work.
>
> **H:** . . . *And* I want you to do it with me. What do you say? You, me, Pilates?
>
> **W:** Bring it on! I mean, not for me! *[both laughing]* Please. I can't even touch my toes!
>
> **H:** But that's the idea. You'll get stronger, you'll get more flexible. All right, you can just watch. Maybe you'll get inspired. And you can work on getting more limber.

Despite their markedly different stages of change, this couple uses humor and mutual understanding to avoid a stalemate. What might have been real resistance on her part is transformed into concern and support, in three ways: 1) He acknowledges that his exercise will affect her, because she will be on her own while he is off riding; 2) He asks an open-ended question (*"What do you mean?"*) rather than accusing her of undermining his goals; and 3) Most crucially, he conveys how important her health is to him by suggesting the easiest of on-ramps—watching him do Pilates, at least until she sees how painless it is—en route to their becoming healthier as a team.

If Your Partner Is a Saboteur

If you are trying to exercise more, and it seems that your partner is sabotaging your efforts to do so, the Principle of Mutual Understanding orients you to several specific strategies that can bring you closer to your goals:

BE AWARE OF THE THREAT YOU MAY BE CREATING. First and foremost, recognize the possibility that your desire to be more active is stirring up feelings of threat and insecurity in your partner. Find ways to encourage connection, and be sensitive to your mate. Recognize, too, that telling your partner about his or her insecurities, without acknowledging your role in generating them, is likely to backfire.

BE SPECIFIC ABOUT YOUR GOALS AND MOTIVATIONS. A way of reducing any sense of threat or discomfort is to clarify for your partner what you are trying to achieve. Uncertainty and ambiguity only add fuel to your partner's sense of vulnerability. For example, one healthy and fit forty-three-year-old woman explained how she wanted to start lifting weights "like a savage," with the vague possibility in mind that she would become very muscular one day. Her real goals were not clear even to her, but by hinting at such an extreme change in her body, she provoked her husband to sabotage any attempts she made to visit the gym.

RECOGNIZE YOUR DIFFERENT STAGES OF CHANGE. If you are way ahead of your partner in the quest to burn a lot of calories, your partner will feel more threatened than if you were at the same starting point and heading in the same direction. This does not mean you need to wait for your partner to catch up to you, but it does mean that your partner's position will need to be acknowledged if you want to cultivate the best possible support for your goals.

FIND WAYS TO STRENGTHEN YOUR PARTNER'S POSITION. If your partner is having difficulty allowing you to be more active, he or she may feel subordinate in the relationship and angry about being put in a one-down position. Resistance will follow. Take steps to restore this imbalance, either by helping your partner to see that your reasons for exercising are not a threat to him or her or the relationship or, better still, by teaming up with your partner while exercising. One woman we watched was able to do this especially well:

> I know we are not in the same place yet when it comes to exercise,
> but if we could find two treadmills side by side at the rec center, then
> we could each go at whatever speeds we wanted but still be together.
> I would love that!

If You Are the Saboteur

If your partner is coming to you for help in incorporating more exercise into his or her daily routine, and is not finding much success in doing so, you may be sabotaging those efforts. The Principle of Mutual Understanding offers you specific guidance as well:

ACKNOWLEDGE THE POSSIBILITY THAT YOUR PARTNER'S EXERCISE MAKES YOU UNCOMFORTABLE. Having a partner who is intent on jump-starting an exercise routine can make you feel insecure about your own appearance and uncertain or even angry about how you figure into your partner's plans. This is a normal and natural (if not always rational) reaction. Pay attention to your feelings when your partner's exercise comes up in your discussions, have an open and honest discussion with your partner about your reactions, and explain your perspective without diminishing it. Voice your concerns, but also offer solutions by giving your partner specific ideas about what he or she might do to help you feel less defensive.

EMBRACE YOUR DIFFERENCES. Recognize that some of the discomfort you are feeling could stem from you and your partner having different goals and agendas when it comes to exercise. There is no inherent problem with this—until you drag your partner down to your lower level of activity. Partners often have different levels and preferences for physical activity, and often differ dramatically in how beneficial they find it for stress reduction and weight management. Make your approach work for you, on your own terms, while encouraging your partner to make the healthiest possible decisions for him- or herself.

KEEP UP. Find ways to benefit from having a healthy partner. As you get beyond feeling threatened by your partner's exercise program, recognize that he or she is effectively creating a new environment that will make it easier for you to be healthier and more active. Take full advantage of this gift, by complementing what he or she is already doing—preparing more vegetables at dinner, for example, or purchasing some hand weights to carry while walking—and join in when your partner heads to the gym or takes a walk around the neighborhood.

THE REASSURANCE TRAP

What are we actually asking for when we say we want our partner's help to exercise more? Our observations suggest that we want to be *motivated and inspired* for what we are trying to accomplish, *and* that we want to be *appreciated and valued* in the relationship so we can feel better about ourselves. Couples fall into the Reassurance Trap because they fail to see that these two needs are fundamentally different.

The first goal (feeling motivated and inspired) has a lot more to do with *behaving* in a certain way—hitting the gym, picking up weights, walking around the neighborhood. But the second goal (feeling appreciated and valued) is more about *feeling* a certain way—wanting to feel capable, competent, confident. Focusing on either need, while neglecting the other, creates more inertia than movement.

It is easy to confuse these two needs—and it's also easy to get the proportions wrong. Offer too much motivation without the proper support (*"I know you can get up in the morning to exercise, but you keep putting it off. What's wrong with you?"*), and your partner may feel like you're "pushing." Offer too much appreciation or support (*"I love you just the way you are! You don't need to change!"*) and your partner may not see the need to change at all. This paradox is the Reassurance Trap—to best support your loved one, you need to offer the right mix of reassurance and motivation. The Principle of Mutual Understanding can help us do that.

Let's take a closer look at how the Reassurance Trap works. The man below says he is not moving enough, and he says he feels bad about it. Neither partner knows it, but his wife is being handed a large and complicated problem, and she assumes that reassurance alone is the balm her husband needs to jump-start his exercise routine.

H: My clothes aren't fitting as well anymore, and I feel unattractive because of it, and so I'd really like to be able to get in shape and just start working out more.

W: Do you know that I love you? Do you know that there is not anything about you that is less attractive to me now than when we first met? And from the time we first met, I was extremely attracted to the way you looked, in addition to your personality.

H: Keep going . . . .

W: But sometimes I feel like you don't realize that it doesn't bother me at all. There's nothing that I would change on you; there's no problem area that I think you have. It's not a problem for me. And sometimes I feel that because you're so insecure about it, that you just maybe don't realize that I feel that way or it doesn't make that much of a difference . . . even if you ended up like the Stay Puft Marshmallow Man, I would still find you incredibly attractive. It would not bother me at all.

What's not to like? Like the Charmers in chapter 5, these partners are offering genuinely kind words, and they provide plenty of heartfelt sympathy for a distressed partner. But by themselves they leave their mates adrift when it comes to actually working out more. You might think that unadulterated praise and encouragement would prompt help-seekers to finally get moving. Surprisingly, however, this approach has two big downsides. First, being praised for who we are and reassured about how we look does have the short-term effect of draining that pool of negative emotion we are feeling when we seek help, while also building solidarity with our partner. But it also rewards us for our passivity. It is almost as if we hear the reassurance and say to ourselves, *"If my partner thinks I look really great just the way I am, without regular exercise, who am I to argue?! I might just stay here on the couch, gain a few more pounds, and then see what she says!"* The second limitation soon becomes clear: reassurance fails to solve the basic problem. We are still not moving enough. The reassurance feels great, but it does not address the gap that exists between our wanting to exercise and our actual level of activity. The real cause of our negative emotions remains in effect.

Other mates go out of their way to avoid this route into the Reassurance Trap but fall into the trap just the same. They downplay the importance of reassurance and focus instead on changing the partner's substandard exercise habits. Like the Taskmasters from chapter 4, these well-intentioned mates really do want the best for the help-seeking partner, but they understand the issue exclusively as a behavioral problem, and their options for changing those behaviors are surprisingly limited. Confronted by a partner who really does want to change their behavior, and who might even be increasingly desperate to do so, these mates tend to be too rigid and strict with the help that they do provide. They hear the help-seeker's frustration, but rather than sympathize with it, they work hard to gain control over it.

> **H:** Well, I'm frustrated. What I think what it is with me is I start doing great, then something gets in the way and I stop going. I don't understand.
>
> **W:** We've talked about this so many times. The thing that gets in the way is that you get burned out. You give up too easily. That's your whole pattern, right there.
>
> **H:** I know. I feel terrible. I feel terrible all the time, every day.
>
> **W:** Then do something about it besides complain about it.
>
> **H:** I know. It's hard, though, and I don't understand why.
>
> **W:** Because you're a big dude. I think you always look in the mirror and you say, "I should be this tight muscular stud." I mean, let's be completely honest.
>
> **H:** No, I don't have to be buff or anything. But 180, 185 is a good weight and I'm over and beyond that. And I don't feel good . . .
>
> **W:** Then you need to do something about it . . . you need to prioritize if these are things you're really upset about.

You might think that some people would appreciate an unsentimental and candid analysis of their unhealthy habits, perhaps even seeing value in the structure and guidance that flows from the "let's be completely honest" vantage point. Some people probably do gain some momentum from this approach, but many others report that it backfires, actually reducing their inclination to get moving again. There is a good reason for this: without any emotional support to soften it, the message arrives as harsh and strident, often leaving the help-seeker to conclude that the partner's affection is contingent upon exercising. The partner becomes the punitive standard-bearer in the relationship, pulling both into the Reassurance Trap—in this instance because reassurance is in such short supply.

The woman in the following couple—let's call her Annie—is concerned that her husband's affection for her depends on her appearance. Annie wants to get back to a regular exercise program and complains because her husband is overly focused on her weight while failing to offer much understanding for her situation.

W: So, basically . . . I want to lose weight.

H: I definitely think you could lose a few pounds.

W: *[with sarcasm]* Oh yeah? Really? That comes as such a shock, because you haven't told me that at all! I mean, are you less attracted to me?

H: Sexually, no. But, when we went to Hermosa [Beach] that one time—I mean, yeah, sometimes your stomach seems really flabby . . . It's one thing if you were working out a lot, but you really aren't making much effort, at least you haven't been.

W: *[hurt]* Well, I'm trying. I know it's a problem, I know it is. I want to exercise, and I'm addressing it now, I feel like that's what should matter . . . . I just want you to appreciate me. How would you feel if I judged you?

H: Did I say—?

W: The "butterball" comments don't go very far to bolster my self-esteem . . . I know you're just being very matter-of-fact and practical, but approaching a sensitive issue with me in that manner, instead of being productive, it ends up being totally counterproductive. It makes me *less* likely to work out—especially if I'm making an effort and you're still making comments, why would I even try?

H: So from now on I should just tell you I love you no matter what?

W: No! You should *act* like you love me no matter what!

You can probably see why this approach doesn't work: these tactics create feelings of guilt, anger, and inadequacy or failure in the person who is trying to change. Help-seekers like Annie are all too aware of the big gap between how much they should exercise and how much they do exercise, and in fact, for Annie, so many negative emotions are churned up when she discusses her weight that the conversation basically shuts down. It is an especially inefficient way to motivate anyone to be more active.

So how can the Principle of Mutual Understanding help couples maneuver their way around the Reassurance Trap? Among the couples implementing this principle successfully, what strikes us most is that recognizing and resolving this issue was not particularly easy for them. There is a "hard-earned" quality to their discussions, in the sense that the resolutions required real thought and effort. Partners in these successful couples seem to have struggled to separate the behavioral and emotional parts of this problem—clear evidence of how deep emotions can run when relationship partners talk about something as personal as their weight and appearance. We are also struck by the intimacy and closeness these couples now radiate as a result of these negotiations.

> **H:** I guess I've pressured you in the past to lose weight. I'm not going
> to pressure you anymore. I love you for who you are. I would
> like to see you at a lighter weight—you know that—but I also
> want you to know that I'm there for you and I'm not going to
> pressure you. It's your choice. I'm going to help you [reach your
> fitness goals] because I think it's important and you could be more
> attractive even though you are still attractive to me. Okay? I love
> you.
> **W:** I love you too.

Like this man, the woman in the example below recognizes the difference between reassuring her partner and underscoring the importance of regular activity. Because she is a bit more passionate about her own exercise than he is about his, her comments clarify for him how she feels about his weight and his approach to exercise.

H: I am paranoid about my appearance and I'm concerned because I know that it's important to you and I don't want to disappoint you. So when I start gaining weight it makes me very concerned because I always feel that's super important to you . . . .

W: The biggest concern that I have is if you don't care. It's not that you're perfect. And maybe it's not that you care that you want to go on the elliptical like I do, but you care that you want to lift weights or run because you love it and it's healthy for you.

H: But when you say that, what I hear is, "She wants me to be muscular, a hard-body."

W: I want you to at least admit that you're not worried that I'm not going to love you or I'm going to love you less because of how you look. That is something I would never do.

H: I know. But it's not important to me to be big and muscular—it's never been who I am. But what I do look to be is just slim. That looks more healthy to me.

W: That's *wonderful* . . . I'm just very concerned about you. If you don't take care of yourself, and if I don't take care of myself, we'll both be dead at too young an age. So it's more about an attitude and a lifestyle than a few pounds.

H: Yeah, I agree. That's why I want to work out in a way that I enjoy it.

Where some partners (like Annie's husband) say or imply, "*If you do not take good care of yourself, I will think less of you,*" this woman is saying, "*I love you unconditionally, and I want us to make our health part of the foundation of our relationship.*" That is a powerful message, because it recognizes her partner's need to feel valued and cared for, while acknowledging his need to stay active and healthy. Ultimately, of course, we all need to move our own muscles to gain the benefits that come from regular exercise. But smart partners like these are more likely to make that happen by validating each other for who they are *and* for who they are exercising to become.

If You or Your Partner Have Fallen into the Reassurance Trap

If you want to exercise more, find yourself struggling a bit in the process, and sense that your partner may be misunderstanding you and your goals, the Principle of Mutual Understanding gives you some options:

ASK FOR WHAT YOU NEED. Be clear about what you are and are not asking for from your partner. Your partner needs clear guidance and direction from you in order to be helpful, and you need to provide your partner with clear feedback about what is and is not working for you. If it is more reassurance you need, ask for that, and express appreciation when it comes your way. If it seems that your partner is misreading your readiness to exercise, help him or her to make the adjustments that will serve you best. And if you feel criticized or misunderstood, offer your partner better alternatives that will help you meet your goals.

DEVELOP SELF-RELIANCE. At the same time, try to not rely too heavily on your partner to get you moving toward your goals. Too much reassurance can make us complacent, whereas overloading our partners with demands to get us moving can prompt a backlash. Take initiative, even if you start off slow with your new exercise routine, and find your motivation within yourself. Ultimately you will prove yourself to be an easier person to help if and when the need does arise.

LISTEN TO WHAT YOUR PARTNER IS SAYING. Research shows that when we are anxious and vulnerable, we tend to think less of ourselves, and also mistakenly assume that our partners share this negative view of us. So, when we approach our partners for help, naturally we believe that they, too, see us as lazy and unmotivated. But more often than not, we are exaggerating our partners' opinions of us, making it out to be worse than it really is and then getting upset because we are not being treated better! Pinning this on your partner is likely to make him or her defensive and uncooperative, so if you approach your partner for help, and end up feeling engulfed by negative experiences, double-check to make sure you are not exaggerating your partner's opinions and recommendations.

If your partner turns to you for help in exercising more but is not moving as much as he or she wants, you might be failing to notice the Reassurance Trap. The Principle of Mutual Understanding suggests some alternatives:

BE THE COACH AND ADVISER, NOT THE JUDGE AND JURY. Remember that if your partner is asking for your help, you have not one but two missions: 1) to provide the right amount of emotional reassurance so that your partner knows that you will be ready and willing to support his or her goals; and 2) to see value in those goals and in the specific steps your partner is taking to reach them. Notice the efforts that your partner is taking to move forward, and when momentum starts to wane, nudge him or her back on track in the most positive and supportive way. Judging and evaluating is not necessary; your partner is already doing enough of this for him- or herself.

ANTICIPATE OBSTACLES AND PROPOSE SMART ALTERNATIVES. While you do want to default to positive forms of support whenever you can, you can still offer thoughtful perspectives on your partner's exercise struggles. Experimental studies demonstrate that anticipating problems and engaging in astute troubleshooting can help people to be more active, beyond simply being told about the beneficial effects of regular exercise. Asking your partner what exercise goal he or she is hoping to accomplish (e.g., going to the gym three times a week) and what benefits this will yield (e.g., feel more fit, less stressed) will bring him or her closer to the goal, *especially if you also encourage your partner to think about the most critical obstacle likely to be encountered and specific ways that obstacle will be circumvented.* For example, having to stay late at work might interfere with your partner's goal of exercising three days a week, but by helping your partner brainstorm ways around that obstacle—trying to get to work early, say, or being sure to exercise the next day—puts a plan in place that keeps the goal in sight.

LET SOMEONE ELSE SET THE STANDARD. As your partner tries to get moving on a consistent basis, you may be inclined to help by making the goal especially clear and concrete. (*"I heard on the radio that we need a minimum of thirty minutes of exercise each day, and so much the better if you can sprint part of the time. How's that working for you?"*) But this puts you in the role of having to be the standard-bearer, undercutting your ability to provide reassurance and support. Rather than become the standard-bearer, let your partner work out his or her own goals, or consider providing your partner with reasonable options from independent authorities; a medical or exercise professional is best, but a well-researched book or website might also work.

KEY POINTS FROM CHAPTER 8

- When one partner asks his or her mate for help and support in exercising more, the mate may feel insecure about his or her own appearance, upset or angry about needing to exercise to keep up, or threatened by the prospects of being in a relationship with a slimmer, sexier person.

- As mates we naturally work to counter these threatening feelings so that we can continue to maintain positive impressions of ourselves, but in the process we may inadvertently resist and undermine our partners' exercise goals. When this happens, we have become *Saboteurs*.

- A second trap is set when mates offer corrective and even well-intentioned feedback without enough emotional reassurance. The feedback registers all too easily as criticism, leaving partners to feel even worse than they already do about their exercise habits. Paradoxically, even a mate's reassurance can prevent the partner from moving more, because this enables the partner to feel good about himself or herself in the short term while leaving the core problem—insufficient activity—unaddressed. These are the two versions of the *Reassurance Trap,* and couples fall into them, as

you can see, when mates provide either too little *or* too much reassurance to the partner seeking to exercise more.

- The Principle of Mutual Understanding helps to resolve the Reassurance Trap, by encouraging mates to see that their help-seeking
partners need, first, the reassurance that will boost esteem and
enable them to experience the relationships as unconditional and
valued resources and, second, recognition and reinforcement for
wanting to exercise more and for taking steps toward specific workout goals. Addressing either aspect of this problem is insufficient,
but providing sensitive doses of emotional *and* behavioral support
maximizes chances for regular, sustained exercise.

PLANNING FOR CHANGE

Each of the statements below describes something that successful couples do to support each partner's efforts to move more. For each one,
consider how well you and your partner engage in this behavior, and
how easy or difficult it will be for the two of you to make any needed
improvements.

1. We each recognize that *we might be putting our partner in a difficult or
   uncomfortable position* when either of us is making changes in our exercise
   habits. We try to avoid reverting to self-protection and resistance, while encouraging mutual connection.

   ____ This is a real strength for us. We do not need to make changes in this
   area.

   ____ We could improve in this area, and we think it will be easy to do so.

   ____ We could improve in this area, but we think it will be difficult to do so.

2. We *recognize that we might be different* in how we want to exercise and
   move more, and we do not use this as an excuse to sabotage each other.

   ____ This is a real strength for us. We do not need to make changes in this
   area.

____ We could improve in this area, and we think it will be easy to do so.
____ We could improve in this area, but we think it will be difficult to do so.

3. We make it very clear to each other that *our relationship is a source of reassurance and unconditional support* when it comes to exercising more.
____ This is a real strength for us. We do not need to make changes in this area.
____ We could improve in this area, and we think it will be easy to do so.
____ We could improve in this area, but we think it will be difficult to do so.

4. We combine reassurance with *validation for our exercise-related goals,* and with *praise and recognition for the specific steps we each take* toward these goals.
____ This is a real strength for us. We do not need to make changes in this area.
____ We could improve in this area, and we think it will be easy to do so.
____ We could improve in this area, but we think it will be difficult to do so.

5. We collaborate so that we can *anticipate the obstacles* we might face when we exercise while also *identifying strategies for overcoming these obstacles* when they arise.
____ This is a real strength for us. We do not need to make changes in this area.
____ We could improve in this area, and we think it will be easy to do so.
____ We could improve in this area, but we think it will be difficult to do so.

6. We *express appreciation* for the support and encouragement that we give each other when we are working to exercise more. We emphasize what we find most valuable in the support we receive.
____ This is a real strength for us. We do not need to make changes in this area.
____ We could improve in this area, and we think it will be easy to do so.
____ We could improve in this area, but we think it will be difficult to do so.

7. We *avoid criticism and insensitive comments* about each other's weight and exercise habits.

    ____ This is a real strength for us. We do not need to make changes in this area.

    ____ We could improve in this area, and we think it will be easy to do so.

    ____ We could improve in this area, but we think it will be difficult to do so.

If you found yourself marking the first answer a lot, then you and your partner clearly appreciate the Principle of Mutual Understanding and have been exploiting that understanding to reinforce each other's efforts to move more.

If your responses tend toward the second answer, then real change is in reach. Now that you understand how the Principle of Mutual Understanding works, you and your partner have a number of great ways to meet your goals for regular exercise, and you are well on your way to working together to make those improvements happen.

If you found yourself often marking the third answer, then you and your partner may understand the Principle of Mutual Understanding but still recognize that making this principle work for you in your own lives will not be easy. Consider reviewing this chapter again with an eye toward identifying just a few concrete steps that you can take today. Collaborate to identify a few good starting points, and then continue collaborating so that you can implement them effectively in your daily lives.

9

Moving More and
Long-Term Commitment

WORKING OUT HOW TO WORK OUT

ROWING UP, TREVOR WAS "the fat kid." He was teased a lot,
picked last for every sport, and had trouble keeping up with
other kids, all of which left emotional wounds that were slow
to heal. By the end of high school he had made the decision to lose
weight and get fit, and by the end of college he had done it, with tremendous effort. He managed to keep the weight off too, through careful attention to what he ate, a rigid schedule at the gym, and bicycling
to and from his job as a video editor. By his late-twenties, he began to
feel confident about his appearance for the first time in his life. He was
in good shape, started wearing tighter clothes, and paid closer attention
to grooming. This was when a friend set him up with Audrey, an associate director of human resources for a pharmaceutical company. They
dated for a year before moving in together, and were married eighteen
months after that.

When they first visited our research rooms, just a few months after
their wedding, Trevor was already worried about his future. His lifestyle

with Audrey was not what it had been when he was a single guy. The bike was gathering dust in the back of the garage, and he had not seen the inside of a gym in a while. After nearly a decade of fitness, he had begun to put on weight again. Looking in the mirror, he started to see echoes of the heavy child he had once been, and the prospect of returning to those days scared him deeply. When we gave them the chance to talk to each other, he tried to express his concerns to Audrey.

> **Trevor:** I think that a lot of my intimacy problems have to do with the way I feel about myself. Because you know I used to be really heavy growing up and then in college I lost quite a bit of weight. When we first started dating, I was a lot thinner than I am now. I guess I stopped exercising and slowly put weight back on, and it's making me feel not as good about myself as I once did.
>
> **Audrey:** Then why don't you exercise anymore?
>
> **Trevor:** It's harder to find the time, but there's no excuse really. I mean, I don't have the space I used to have.
>
> **Audrey:** What about your bike?
>
> **Trevor:** Yeah, I should bike, you're right. Before we were dating, I used to come home, ride my bike or whatever, but when I started seeing you three, four times a week, I'd come home and shower instead. I guess I gradually worked my way out of my regimen and I never picked it up again. I think that has a lot to do with how I feel about myself. And I'm not too happy with the way I am right now.

Trevor is haunted by the ghosts of his past. He is still far from the heavy kid he was growing up, but as he looks ahead on the path that he and Audrey seem to be on, Trevor sees the hard-won gains he has made in his physical fitness slipping away. The result is a lot of negative emotion: guilt over his failure to keep exercising, shame about his recent weight gain, and anxiety about what may happen if he does not make a change.

Audrey was worried about Trevor too, but not for the same reasons. An attractive woman a couple of years older than Trevor, Audrey did not have to work very hard to stay slim. Exercise was not her thing; she had never been tempted to join a gym. She cared less about fitness than about physical appearance, and she was concerned about the changes she was noticing in the handsome man she had married. In our research rooms, she tried to understand exactly what was bothering him.

Audrey: Do you think that your beard has anything to do with it?

Trevor: *[laughing]* The beard is just a fling. It'll probably be off in a month. It doesn't weigh too much.

Audrey: But it's a physical thing. Do you think you grew the beard to hide behind?

Trevor: No.

Audrey: Okay, I was just asking. What about your clothes? Do your clothes have anything to do with it?

Trevor: *[puzzled]* You mean how I'm outgrowing all my old clothes?

Audrey: No, I mean how you wear clothes that don't necessarily match.

Trevor: *[speechless]* . . .

Audrey: Wait, aren't we talking about your physical appearance?

Trevor: My body. We are talking about my body, my physical body, not my style.

Audrey: Oh, I thought you meant your physical look.

Trevor: *[slowly, patiently]* I think a lot of the way I feel about my body comes from the memory of being fat. I got to be in pretty good shape. I want to feel attractive.

Audrey: Do you think you're not as attractive because you're going bald? Does that bother you?

Trevor: Are you like—is that supposed to be funny?

Audrey: I'm just asking!

As she says, she is just asking. But instead of deepening her understanding of the challenges her husband is facing, Audrey's questions only reveal their failure to connect. Trevor has just told her what he thinks the problem is—he wants to get back in shape. Coming so soon after that disclosure, Audrey's questions about Trevor's wardrobe and grooming strike him not as genuine expressions of interest, but as attempts to change the subject. The more Trevor tries to stay focused on his plan to get more exercise, the more Audrey's resistance to the idea becomes clear.

Audrey: So is that your only solution—to join a gym?

Trevor: Why? What do you have against me joining a gym?

Audrey: I'm just asking! I look at the financial aspect of it.

Trevor: I will pay for it . . .

Audrey: But how long are they locking you in for? That's my only question.

Trevor: It's per month.

Audrey: Are you sure?

Trevor: Yeah.

Audrey: You called and asked?

Trevor: Yes.

Audrey: And they said per month for thirty-six months?

Trevor: If it was, I wouldn't do it, but no.

Audrey: If that'll make you happy, then do that.

By this point in their conversation, all Trevor has done is express an interest in getting more exercise, something that has been hard for him to do in recent years. He has not actually joined a gym or taken any other action. Nevertheless Audrey interrogates him as if he were the prime suspect in a television cop drama. So Trevor's question back to her is reasonable: what *does* she have against his joining the gym? At first she seems concerned about the financial commitment that

gym memberships often entail, but even after Trevor assures her—
repeatedly—that he can join without a lengthy contract, she does not
seem comforted. She manages a halfhearted *"If that'll make you happy, then
do that,"* but cannot bring herself to declare her enthusiastic support.

The consequences of their inability to see eye to eye emerged when
they returned to our research rooms two years later. Trevor had gained
more weight over that time, and when we offered them a chance to talk
together, their conversation began on a familiar note.

> **Trevor:** I was thinking . . .
>
> **Audrey:** Oh no, thinking again!
>
> **Trevor:** . . . about joining a gym.
>
> **Audrey:** You've been talking about joining a gym forever.
>
> **Trevor:** I know. It's a minor expense, but it's convenient. After work, I
> could just go to the gym and work out for an hour, and we'd be
> home at the same time. Remember? When I was working out and
> in shape, I had a better attitude toward everything—you, myself,
> everyone. You know what I'm saying?

As far as Trevor's getting more exercise, they are exactly where
they began two years before. It is easy to imagine that, between their
visits to our lab, they have had repeated variations of this same conversation over and over, with Trevor expressing his negative feelings
about himself and his powerful desire to get back in shape, and Audrey
withdrawing or expressing mild resistance. Clearly, it is not a conversation that gets them any closer to a plan for action. They both care
about each other's well-being, so what keeps them in this frustrating
cycle? The answer became clearer during this visit, when Audrey, who
now was pregnant with their first child, started to open up about her
concerns for their future.

> **Trevor:** If I joined a gym, I'm sure I would go.
>
> **Audrey:** Even after the baby is born?

Trevor: Yeah, that's something we'd need to discuss. How do you feel about that?

Audrey: I've never been a big gym fan myself.

Trevor: I know. You don't like to sweat.

Audrey: Not just that. I just mean as far as people joining gyms.

Trevor: Why? As far as people joining and they don't go?

Audrey: They tend not to go or their schedules change and it's just inconvenient to go. What if I get a job and you have to be in charge of the baby? How are you going to go to the gym after work?

Trevor: I think we would cross that bridge when we get to it.

Audrey: But if you join a gym, you can't just join for a couple months and then quit. They lock you in for a year. The baby is coming in three months.

Finally Audrey has expressed the source of her resistance: she fears that Trevor's commitment to a gym (and, by implication, to his own health) will take priority over his commitment to her and their baby. For Trevor, getting to the gym and dividing child care are completely separate issues, and he is fine postponing the child-care conversation until after the baby is born. For Audrey, the two issues are linked. She recognizes that every hour Trevor spends at the gym is an hour he is not at home. As she looks three months into their future, she wants to know that Trevor will be there when she needs him. Audrey cares about Trevor's weight issues, but she cares more about being her husband's first priority. Trevor does not recognize how his intentions to join a gym threaten his wife's security, so all he registers is her reluctance to support his health.

Trevor: It seems to me that you are looking for an excuse for me not to do it. *[joking]* Are you afraid I'm going to get good-looking and go after some other girl?

Audrey: *[sarcastically]* Yeah, that's it. *[seriously]* No, all I'm trying to do is postpone the gym thing till we know what's going on with me

and my job, that's all. I'm thinking that rather than you getting
locked into something—say I do get a job in August and you're in
charge of the kid, you know. I'm trying to just—look, I don't care
if you join a gym. If it makes you feel better, that's fine.

Trevor: I told you I would pay for it.

Audrey: I'm not worried about that. I'm just trying to look at other
ways for you to exercise, something you can do when you're at
home. Or postpone the whole thing until we know where we'll
be after the baby. I'm just trying to see when the best time for you
to join would be. Wait until we know what's going on, or go now?
I'm trying to think about other angles.

Trevor began this conversation, like all of their other conversations
about exercise, with one question: how can he get to the gym regularly?
They never come up with an answer, because Audrey has other questions that come first for her. Is this even the right time in their lives
to make a serious lifestyle change? If there is a choice between caring for children and working out, which commitment takes priority?
Will Trevor's desire to get to the gym interfere with Audrey's ability to
pursue her career? Audrey loves her husband, but she sees his need for
exercise as competing with her needs for support at home. As long as
they both accept this premise, they are trapped in an awful bind: the
more they are devoted to their growing family, the more they will tend
to prevent each other from pursuing activities that keep each of them
healthy. Indeed, that is where Trevor and Audrey seem to have stopped,
and nothing in this conversation offers much hope that Trevor will be
able to get any more exercise after their baby is born than he has been
getting in the years prior to their baby's arrival.

The challenges that Trevor and Audrey face integrating exercise
into their lives are not unique to new parents. The desire for a healthier
lifestyle always raises broader issues for couples, because a commitment
to fitness is never the only commitment that couples make. Yes, most of
us want our partners to be active and healthy, but we also want them to

be supportive and available. We want our partners to take care of themselves, but we also want them to take care of us and of our relationships. When these goals are viewed as competing with each other, partners like Trevor and Audrey find that the more they love each other and are devoted to their relationship, the harder it is to integrate physical fitness into their lives. A great relationship may end up working against our health instead of supporting it.

The way out of this dilemma is to *question the premise that a commitment to fitness competes with a commitment to the relationship*. On the contrary, the Principle of Long-Term Commitment suggests that, over the course of a relationship, these goals are intertwined. If we want long lives with our partners, then committing to our relationships requires committing to our partners' health.

When we applied this principle to eating right in chapter 6, we emphasized how our love for our partners can help to keep wavering dieters on the right track. The same idea applies to exercise, in that the desire for a long, healthy life can absolutely be part of what pulls a loving partner off the couch and onto a bike. But exercise, as we have seen in the last two chapters, also raises some new issues, like how to make room for physical activity in a busy schedule. In this chapter, we will show how taking a long-term perspective on our commitments offers ways for our health goals and our relationship goals to reinforce and support each other, rather than conflict. But first we will describe why weaving exercise into the fabric of our lives can be so challenging for many of us.

EXERCISE OVER THE LIFE SPAN: WHAT KIDS KNOW AND ADULTS FORGET

Many adults complain—accurately—that they are not getting enough exercise. Yet you rarely hear young children with the same complaint (*"Mommy, I have got to get to the jungle gym more often."*). Children are regularly set loose in parks and playgrounds. The elementary-school day is structured around recess and physical education. In secondary school, youths drag heavy backpacks full of books down corridors and up stairways to get from class to class. Exercise is not an accessory to the routines of childhood; it is an essential part of what it means to be a child.

And then what happens? Research that has tracked levels of physical activity across the life span has been as consistent as its results have been dramatic: physical activity plummets after childhood. In one study that used accelerometers to track people's movements throughout the day, 42 percent of children between the ages of six and eleven met recommended levels of activity. In stark contrast, only 8 percent of adolescents between twelve and eighteen reached that level, and less than 5 percent of adults did. Study after study finds that physical activity continues to decline as we age.

What changes after childhood can help us understand the drastic shift in the amount of exercise across our lives? Research on this question has confirmed roles for all the familiar suspects: busier schedules, competing obligations, and reduced access to equipment (it is easier to find a park than a gym, and parks are free). But a persistent, and perhaps surprising, theme across this work is that, as we get older, the decision to exercise becomes more closely tied to our relationships.

The social aspects of exercise seem to emerge in adolescence, just when levels of exercise begin to drop. For example, in one study that asked fifth- and sixth-grade children why they engaged in physical activity, the only answer that predicted how much they actually exercised was how much they said they enjoyed exercising. Active children moved more because they liked being active. Two years later, however, interviews with those same children, now in seventh and eighth grade, revealed that their own enjoyment of exercise no longer predicted how much they exercised. By junior high school, their *activity levels were more strongly associated with whether or not their friends were exercising.*

And the battle just heats up from there. After college, young adults describe greater feelings of self-efficacy when it comes to exercise. That is, they know how much exercise they want, and where they might get it. Yet they are even less physically active than college students, because they perceive greater barriers to exercise as well. Again, research suggests that many of those barriers are associated with relationships, like competing obligations to partners, spouses, and children. Older adults, in contrast, report fewer barriers to exercise, but nevertheless still exercise less on average than younger adults. It is possible that, by the time couples face empty nests and opportunities for exercise might become available, older adults' priorities have shifted permanently, and exercise remains a secondary concern. Indeed, there is evidence that over time sedentary behavior becomes a habit that is extremely hard to break.

Because our level of physical activity is wrapped up in our social world, when we choose relationships, we are choosing lifestyles as well. If we have athletic friends and active hobbies, exercise may become an enduring part of our identities as adults. If the people we socialize with spend their time in other ways, then we are more likely to leave exercise behind as we spend more time with them. To the extent that we select our romantic partners from within our social networks, our intimate relationships often serve to crystallize those patterns of physical activity (or inactivity). For a couple whose routine has never included regular exercise, participating in the relationship therefore reinforces sedentary habits. For such couples, exercise becomes something separate from the relationship, another chore to add to their already lengthy lists.

It doesn't have to be this way. The Principle of Long-Term Commitment reminds us that setting up a "competition" between good health and the needs of our relationships is an illusion. If we love our partners and want them to stick around through old age, then our commitment to them *requires* a commitment to their health, and to our own. Rather than competing with our relationships, physical activity can *nurture* our relationships, especially when we remember what most of us knew as children: being physically active is a way to live in the world, and can be a way to live in our relationships as well.

In the rest of this chapter, we will explain how shifting to a long-term perspective can help partners who are struggling to balance their commitments to each other with their commitments to an active lifestyle. Toward this goal, we will offer suggestions for letting go of the three obstacles that get in the way of couples trying to strike this balance:

1. The *Guilty Conscience Problem* stems from the assumption that exercising is selfish, something partners do for themselves and not for the relationship.
2. In the *Moving Target Trap,* conflicts arise when partners have different goals when it comes to exercise.
3. *Burnout* is the frustration that some partners feel when their support and encouragement fail to lead to positive changes in their partners' habits.

In each case, we will find that what can look like mutually exclusive choices in the short term are often compatible over the course of a long-term commitment.

WHEN IS EXERCISING SELFISH? THE GUILTY CONSCIENCE PROBLEM

No partners are identical, so the longer a relationship lasts, the more inevitable it is that couples encounter times when they have conflicting needs and desires. The tension between Trevor and Audrey is a textbook example: he wanted to make time for the gym, and Audrey wanted to preserve his time for supporting her and their baby. Their disagreement was about how to reconcile their different priorities.

When it comes to exercise, we often see partners struggling with similar conflicts within themselves. In these cases, individual partners feel multiple competing desires at the same time. On the one hand, they know that they should be exercising and taking better care of their physical fitness. On the other hand, they prioritize their relationships and are reluctant to accept any distracting obligations. These partners view working out as self-indulgent, and therefore something that a truly devoted partner should resist. The fact that they feel any conflict at all about exercising becomes a source of anxious questions: Am I being selfish? Do I love my partner enough? Which comes first, my relationship or me?

Resisting exercise for fear of threatening the relationship is a sign of the *Guilty Conscience Problem*. Among the traps that prevent people from being more active, this one is particularly insidious, because it gets its power from partners' commitment to their relationship. The more devoted they are to each other, the more partners trapped by this problem have an excuse not to pursue the exercise they need. For partners who have never been very physically active and might be looking for reasons to avoid exercise, this one is pretty appealing, because it casts the failure to get exercise as something noble (*"I love my partner too much to take care of myself"*). Who could judge someone for loving a partner too much?

The wife in the next couple is clearly struggling with the Guilty Conscience Problem. She still wants it all—time to exercise, time to study for her law degree, and time to cuddle on the couch with her new husband—and the fact that she cannot do all three leaves her feeling inadequate.

> **W:** I think about it every day—okay, I'm going to do this. And then I don't do it, and so I feel like a big lardo. And now I just kind of feel bad because I'm not doing anything, you know?
>
> **H:** Do you feel any of it is my fault?
>
> **W:** No. I think part of the problem is that I feel guilty, like I should be using that time for us to do something instead of to go exercise. You know, that's an hour just getting to the gym and back, and I spend like an hour there. That's time I feel I should have been spending at home with you.
>
> **H:** What if we spend time exercising together?
>
> **W:** Yeah, see, that's the problem. I enjoy the Rollerblading; you don't like to Rollerblade. You don't really like to bike ride either, so I don't know which one you could do.

H: Well, don't feel obligated to spend time with me. I mean, I want
you to spend time with me, but your time at the gym would also
give me time to study, so don't feel like I'd just be sitting at home
doing nothing.

This wife is trapped. She knows she needs more exercise, and has
lots of activities (going to the gym, Rollerblading, bike riding) that she
would enjoy doing. At the same time, she knows that time spent on
any of these activities would take her away from her husband, whom
she already does not see enough. Her guilt arises from the conflict
between these desires, but notice that her husband does not reinforce
her feelings. On the contrary, he supports his wife's desire to get to the
gym, and assures her that he could occupy himself perfectly well in her
absence. The tension she feels lies entirely within her, and it stems from
her own assumption that getting fit and being healthy is something she
would be doing for herself and not for the relationship. To avoid being a
bad partner, she avoids exercising, but the result is just a different kind of
negative experience (feeling "like a big lardo").

The guilt that some partners feel when they contemplate exercising alone makes sense from a short-term perspective. On any one day,
an hour spent at the gym is one hour less to watch television, do dishes,
or catch up with our partners. If one day is all you are thinking about,
then time spent on exercise does seem like taking time away from the
relationship. Yet the Principle of Long-Term Commitment reminds us
that the measure of a relationship is not how we spend any one day, but
how we plan for a lifetime of days. Across weeks, months, and years, it is
easier to imagine finding room for going to the gym one night, doing
dishes the next, and catching up in bed later. Thus, keeping a long-term
perspective in mind offers couples some flexibility in adjusting their
schedules to include exercise.

If You or Your Partner Suffer from the Guilty Conscience Problem

If you or your partner have been worried that exercising makes you less devoted to your relationship, here are some concrete strategies for soothing a guilty conscience:

TREAT EXERCISE AS AN INVESTMENT IN THE FUTURE. Many working couples set aside a portion of their monthly income toward retirement accounts. When it comes to financial matters, they are perfectly willing to forgo the pleasures that the extra money might buy them in the present, so that they may afford comfortable lives in the future. Treat exercise and fitness the same way. An hour that one partner spends at the gym tonight takes time that might have been spent together, but it is also an investment in the active, healthy life that both partners want to enjoy as they get older.

EXPRESS INTEREST IN EACH OTHER'S HEALTH. When our partners confess to feeling guilty about taking care of themselves, sometimes all they need is a little reassurance that we care about their well-being, and that we appreciate all they are doing to be healthy. The husband in our example leans in this direction when he insists that he "has no trouble" with his wife's spending time at the gym without him. But imagine how much more powerful his support would be if he expressed not only *willingness* to accommodate her schedule, but also genuine enthusiasm for her moves toward physical fitness. For example, he might have said, *"Honey, I hear you when you say you feel guilty, but seriously? I want you to go to the gym when you can. I need you healthy for me, for our kids, and for our grandkids. Whatever you do to keep fit is a gift to me. Guilty about going to the gym? I thank you for doing it!"*

TRADE ALONE TIME. When the wife in our example thinks about working out, she feels guilty for more than one reason. Not only would she be taking time from the relationship, but she would be getting exercise while her husband was not. She has the upper hand in that arrangement, but it's not a fair division of benefits, and even advantaged partners are less satisfied with their relationships when they perceive them to be unfair. In the short term, these kinds of inequitable situations are unavoidable. Parents may find that the only way one partner can get time to exercise is if the other partner stays home to provide child care. In the long term, however, the sting of unfairness can be softened when partners make explicit plans to ensure that both partners get what they need. In our example, the husband might have eased his partner's mind if he had assured her that he planned to find time to play basketball with friends on the weekends. The more that both partners see the distribution of time for exercise as fair, the less room there is for guilty feelings to get in the way of actually getting that exercise.

THE MOVING TARGET TRAP: WHO DECIDES HOW MUCH EXERCISE IS ENOUGH?

For the large and growing segment of the adult population that does not exercise regularly, getting started is the hardest part. The partners of individuals who are just beginning exercise routines generally support their desire for a more active lifestyle. Yet sometimes they disagree about the specific goals their mates have set. They have read the headlines about the ideal level of exertion an adult needs to ward off heart disease. They have heard that an individual gets maximum benefit from reaching a specific heart rate and maintaining that heart rate for a specific length of time. Ambitious for their loved ones, these well-meaning partners figure that, if their mates are going to pursue more exercise, they might as well pursue the level of exercise that does the most for their health. Immediately.

With visions of an active partner in mind, and a strong desire to be a source of encouragement, they urge their partners toward different, and higher, standards for exercise than their partners have set for themselves. These partners are raising the bar for what a good workout entails, hoping to motivate greater effort from their less-active mates. Unfortunately, the result of this well-intentioned encouragement can often be to dampen the enthusiasm of the person contemplating a change, rather than to spark it.

We call this the *Moving Target Trap*: when one partner sets a goal that might be within reach, and the other partner, like Lucy holding the football for Charlie Brown, moves the goal to where it may be impossible to reach. Being on the receiving end of this sort of encouragement, as Charlie Brown learned over and over, is demoralizing, and makes that all-important first step harder to take.

The wife in the next example is caught in the Moving Target Trap, and her husband is the one keeping her there. At the time they had the conversation we observed, her husband was going to the gym several times a week after work, but she was on a different schedule and could not join him. As a result, she was getting no regular exercise at all, and knew she was doing her body no favors.

> **W:** I feel like a lazy bum and I want to be healthier. When I don't exercise, I feel fat and gross. When I exercise, I feel like I could conquer the world.
>
> **H:** So do that *all the time*. When we're watching TV, you should be jogging in place.
>
> **W:** Well, what I want is to be able to keep running until I get to like forty minutes.
>
> **H:** Forty minutes!? That's not exercise. You have to go for at least an hour. That's moderate exercise. No, that's not even moderate . . . it's light.
>
> **W:** Well, it makes you sweat. I was sweating.
>
> **H:** *[unimpressed]* It doesn't raise your heart rate as much as it's supposed to.

This wife knows what she wants to accomplish and she expresses it directly: to go from no exercise at all to running for forty minutes at a stretch. That's a concrete and explicit goal, and given her schedule and habits, it won't be easy to reach. Yet, as ambitious as it may seem to her, this husband responds as if her target were not high enough. Ignoring the target she has set for herself, he urges her toward loftier exercise goals ("*You have to go for at least an hour*"), as if she were already running forty minutes, as opposed to still just thinking about it. There is a disconnect because they are concerned about different things: she is focused on the gap between where she is and where she would like to be, while he is focused on the gap between what she is aiming for and what he thinks she needs to get maximum benefit from exercise.

We discussed a similar problem in chapter 6 when we described the Dreamer, someone whose goals for weight loss are so unrealistic that they interfere with taking even one step. In that case, the person seeking change was the one setting the unrealistic goal. In the Moving Target Trap, the person seeking change sets a realistic goal, but has a partner who dismisses or ignores that goal, proposing a more difficult one. In both cases, the result is to reduce the likelihood that the partner seeking change will develop a plan and enact it: *From my position on the couch, the idea of jogging around the block might be worth discussing, but if my partner insists I train for a marathon, I may just forget the whole thing and grab the remote.*

Much like the Guilty Conscience Problem, the Moving Target Trap arises from a short-term perspective on exercise. The husband in our previous example believes that his wife's goal of running forty minutes is incompatible with his advice to run for at least an hour, and so pressures her to abandon one goal for the other. A long-term perspective, however, reminds us that we usually pursue many different goals as we mature. First we aim for the easier ones, and then we take on the harder ones. The wife in our example, currently doing no running at all, could easily aim for forty minutes of running, and then, having reached her target, push toward an hour. Our capacity for exercise, like a relationship, evolves over time. What looks like a moving target from a short-term perspective is just a series of potential accomplishments from the perspective of a long-term commitment to exercise.

If You Have Been Setting a Moving Target Trap for Your Partner

If you have been inadvertently catching your partner in a Moving Target Trap, appreciating the Principle of Long-Term Commitment offers several suggestions for directing your encouragement in more productive ways:

TAILOR EXERCISE ADVICE TO YOUR PARTNER. When it comes to exercise, one size definitely does not fit all. The recommendations that make headlines apply to the average healthy individual, but your partner has unique preferences and capabilities. Rather than jumping in with advice and criticism, you might start by asking a few questions, like:

> What does physical fitness look like for you?
> What kinds of exercise do you prefer?
> What makes getting exercise hard for you?
> What can I do to help?

If your partner is contemplating a lasting change of lifestyle, that's a good place to begin. Meeting the standard recommendations for daily activity levels can come later.

LET YOUR PARTNER CHOOSE A COMFORTABLE LEVEL OF INTENSITY. How hard does your partner need to exercise? One approach to answering this question is to push your partner toward the maximum level of intensity that he or she can sustain, making every workout a stress test. The problem with this approach is that working out harder than is comfortable feels bad. Not everyone likes to be exhausted, and not everyone agrees with "no pain, no gain." When working out is uncomfortable, people are less likely to stick with it, especially if they have not already developed regular exercise habits.

A second approach is to let your partner choose whatever level of intensity feels right for him or her. The good news about this second approach is that, given the freedom, most people who exercise naturally gravitate toward the recommended levels of intensity for their body types. More important, when people choose their own level, they report more pleasure with exercise and are more likely to continue exercising over time. So the aim of your support and encouragement should be to get your partner moving; your partner turns out to be the best person to decide how much and how hard.

REMEMBER THAT ANYTHING IS BETTER THAN NOTHING. If your partner is inactive, your most important task is to get him or her off the couch. So don't raise the bar—lower it. Does your partner complain that thirty minutes of walking sounds like too much time? Try ten minutes. Try five minutes. The hardest bridge to cross is the one between no exercise and any exercise, and that is the one that makes the greatest long-term difference to your partner's health. Do whatever you can to help your partner take that first, hardest step and then keep taking that step day after day. One wife who understood this expressed it perfectly in our research rooms:

> I don't necessarily have to go to the gym for an hour and half because that's not going to fit into my time frame. I just can't do that right now, but there's so many other things I could do to feel better about myself, so that's what I'm going to do. Taking Justin for a walk, going for a little thirty-minute walk or jog—something is better than nothing, right?

BURNOUT: WHEN CARING GETS TOO HARD

Stick with it. That's good advice for exercise and good advice for supporting a partner. But, just as keeping to a regular exercise routine proves difficult for many people, maintaining support for our partners can be difficult too. Real change can be slow, and real progress is not always steady. Our partners may achieve genuine gains for a while and then fall back into old habits. As we watch them struggle to move more and improve their health, how much support are we expected to provide? What happens when the partners we are supporting are not getting anywhere?

Faced with a loved one whose efforts to get healthier have stalled, it is easy to get frustrated. Supportive partners know what their mates have to do to get healthier, and as a result they may have difficulty understanding why their mates don't just get with the program. People who are accustomed to seeing results when they put their minds to something are especially prone to feeling discouraged when their efforts to support their partners do not meet with similar results. After repeatedly trying and failing to make a difference, they may begin to doubt the value of their efforts. None of this feels good. Reluctant to experience frustration over and over, some partners lose faith and gradually withdraw their support altogether.

Psychologists have coined the term *learned helplessness* to describe how people with no control over a situation stop trying to effect change. When it comes to providing support, a more common term is *Burnout*. Caregivers who experience burnout talk about feeling depleted, as if they have given all that they have to give. The result is uninterest in providing additional care. In the couples that visit our research rooms, burnout often expresses itself as impatience with a partner's lack of progress. We discussed impatience back in chapter 6 when we described the Now-or-Never Problem. There, we explained that partners can give up on themselves when they fail to achieve their health goals as quickly as they had hoped. Burnout is a related idea, but it happens when we give up on our partners.

You can hear the impatience in this next husband. Both times this couple visited our research rooms, the wife chose to discuss her weight gain and the challenges she faced trying to manage it. On their first visit, her husband leapt enthusiastically into the support role. He was quick to offer reassurance, and was free with helpful suggestions about ways they might weave more physical activity into their lives. Two years later, the problem she chose to discuss had not changed, but his behavior had. It was clear that she had not made much progress toward her fitness goals, and his frustration was palpable.

> **W:** Well, I'm bummed.
>
> **H:** I know you're bummed. You always say you're bummed. You always say you're overweight, but you don't stick to anything.
>
> **W:** I don't know. I think what it is with me is I start doing good, then I do bad. I don't understand.
>
> **H:** I do understand, and I've told you a million times.
>
> **W:** What?
>
> **H:** You don't—you choose not to listen to me.
>
> **W:** Something throws me off.
>
> **H:** Something that throws you off is that you've never, ever, in your entire life stuck with a program, and it's become a habit. You do it, do it, do it; then you get tired out and you're done. That's the whole thing. You have to plan a daily routine that you're going to stick to. You can't count on me. I can't be responsible. I feel responsible for the things that you do, and I shouldn't.

This wife begins their discussion feeling bummed. Nothing her husband has to say seems likely to improve her mood. Whereas she appears open to a discussion about her problems sticking with exercise, he makes his opinion clear that the time for such a discussion is long past. Instead, he has concluded that her failures are the result of her own character flaws (*"You've never, ever, in your entire life stuck with a program"*). He is convinced that he offered her a way forward and she squandered it (*"You choose not to listen to me"*). He feels he has no choice but to wash his hands of her problems (*"I can't be responsible"*). This is a man who feels helpless to help his partner and so has decided it is no longer his job—all classic signs of burnout. The irony in this case is that she is clearly frustrated and feeling helpless too. The fact that he blames her for not making progress keeps him on opposite sides from her, but they are actually banging their heads against the same wall.

By now you can probably see the culprit: all this frustration is another result of short-term thinking. Partners want to see each other change, or at least see some return on their investment of support, and so they get frustrated and threaten to withdraw when they don't see change soon enough. Expressing frustration can be a last-ditch effort to motivate the partner, sort of an ultimatum (*"Play by my rules or I'm taking my ball and going home!"*). Generally, this is not a successful strategy, because it places an added emotional burden on the partner who may be overwhelmed already. Imagine how the person struggling to get exercise might respond to a partner's ultimatum: *I already know I need more exercise and I am finding it nearly impossible, now I have to worry about your feelings as well?!?* A relationship that partners hope will be a source of reliable support and comfort becomes an additional source of threat instead. No one is helped by this.

If short-term thinking contributes to burnout, then appreciating the Principle of Long-Term Commitment can vaccinate us against burnout by relieving us of the need to expect or demand short-term results from our partners. Thinking about physical activity as a lifelong process offers our partners the space to go slow, to make mistakes, and to try again. Of course, partners who wish to change have to take that first step eventually. But the silver lining of procrastination is that, if that first step did not happen today, tomorrow offers another chance to get it right. It is never too soon to get started, but from a long-term perspective it is never too late either. There's a new opportunity to seize every day, and this is as true for the person seeking change as it is for the supporting partner.

If You Are Experiencing Burnout

When you are feeling frustrated and impatient with your slow-moving partner, here are some suggestions for staying engaged and avoiding burnout:

TEAM UP AGAINST THE PROBLEM. Most likely, you and your partner are in the same boat: you both want to see your partner moving more and getting fit. If your partner is not making the progress you would like to see, it is worth remembering that this is probably as frustrating and confusing to your partner as it is to you. So, do not take your partner's failures personally. Resist the urge to point fingers or assign blame. Instead, unite with your partner. The two of you can be a team, working together to identify and overcome the challenges that are getting in the way of your partner's health. The husband in our example missed an easy opportunity to take this approach. When his wife confessed that she did not understand what throws her off her exercise routine, instead of berating her ("*I've told you a million times*"), he could have taken her side:

> I think you're right. I know how much you want to be more active, but something clearly does throw you off. I'll admit that it has been frustrating for me to see you trying so hard without much to show for it—I can only imagine how frustrating it must be for you. So let's try to figure it out together. Once we name the problem, I know that we can tackle it.

Maybe this approach would have identified a path toward lasting change in her levels of physical activity. But even if it did not, it would have at least united them against frustration, instead of allowing the frustration to get between them.

TRY SOMETHING NEW. If you plan to spend the rest of your life, or even a good portion of your life, with your partner, then giving up is not really an option. If your partner is not going away, then your partner's health issues are not going to go away either. So instead of giving up, get creative. If your partner has been working out alone, you might suggest enrolling in a class with other people. If exercising in a gym has lost its flavor, you can offer a hike or a bike ride outdoors. Staying creative for our partners communicates two valuable messages to them. First, it says that there are options for getting fit that they have not yet tried, and that points them toward hope instead of hopelessness. Second, and just as important, it says that *you* have not given up on them, that you are still engaged and confident in their capacity to change. That's a message your partner needs to hear.

REMEMBER THAT YOU DO NOT HAVE TO SOLVE YOUR PARTNER'S PROBLEMS. One source of burnout is the sense of having failed as a support provider. "*If my support were more effective,*" thinks the burned-out partner, "*then my mate would not still be struggling with this problem.*" No one enjoys feeling like a failure, so this way of thinking tends to lead to the shifting blame onto the partner and withdrawing from the supportive role.

But this way of thinking assumes a narrow definition of what it means to provide effective support. Certainly it can be very supportive to solve our partners' problems, but this is far from the only function that supporting our partners can serve. Even if it does not touch the problem at all, our support can communicate love and confidence in the relationship. Supporting our partners through problems can offer perspective by saying: "*Yes, we are facing a challenge right now, but the challenge does not define us. Our relationship is bigger than the challenges we face.*" In many cases, our partners may not even want us to solve their problems; they may just want to understand themselves better or be reminded that they are not alone. Adopting this wider view of the functions of support opens up a range of ways to define success, and reminds the supportive partner of all the ways they can make a big difference in their partner's life.

KEY POINTS FROM CHAPTER 9

- If exercise is not part of a relationship from the start, then the demands of fitness can be perceived as competing with the demands of the relationship, and research suggests that this is what happens for many people.

- The Principle of Long-Term Commitment reminds us that the competition between the demands of physical fitness and the demands of our relationships is illusory. Over the course of a lifetime together, our commitment to our partners *requires* a commitment to their health and fitness.

- Partners trapped by short-term thinking can fall into the trap of viewing their own efforts to be active as self-centered distractions from the relationship (the *Guilty Conscience Problem*), but a long-term perspective can remind couples that time spent on fitness today is an investment that pays off in a higher quality of life together in the future.

- Partners focused on short-term changes in physical activity sometimes set goals for their partners that are higher and harder to reach than the goals those partners set for themselves (the *Moving Target Trap*). A long-term perspective highlights the importance of getting started with exercise at a level that is comfortable and sustainable.

- When the partner in the support role gets frustrated with a mate that is failing to make progress, the result can be frustration and a desire to withdraw support that seems to be ineffective (*Burnout*). A long-term perspective reminds supportive partners that giving up is not an option, and that supporting our partners can have lasting benefits even if it does not solve their problems right away.

PLANNING FOR CHANGE

This final section invites you to think about how you and your partner are exploiting your long-term commitment right now. Each of the statements below describes something that successful couples do to support each partner's efforts to get enough exercise. For each one, consider how well you and your partner engage in this behavior, and how easy or difficult it will be for the two of you to make any needed improvements.

1. We recognize that the time we spend on physical activities and exercise is an *investment in a shared future together*.

   ____ This is a real strength for us. We do not need to make changes in this area.

   ____ We could improve in this area, and we think it will be easy to do so.

   ____ We could improve in this area, but we think it will be difficult to do so.

2. We express *genuine interest* in each other's health and fitness.

   ____ This is a real strength for us. We do not need to make changes in this area.

   ____ We could improve in this area, and we think it will be easy to do so.

   ____ We could improve in this area, but we think it will be difficult to do so.

3. We allocate time for exercise *fairly*.

   ____ This is a real strength for us. We do not need to make changes in this area.

   ____ We could improve in this area, and we think it will be easy to do so.

   ____ We could improve in this area, but we think it will be difficult to do so.

4. We encourage each other to select *comfortable and sustainable* levels of exercise intensity.

   ____ This is a real strength for us. We do not need to make changes in this area.

   ____ We could improve in this area, and we think it will be easy to do so.

   ____ We could improve in this area, but we think it will be difficult to do so.

5. We *unite as a team* to overcome any obstacles to getting the exercise we need.

   ____ This is a real strength for us. We do not need to make changes in this area.

   ____ We could improve in this area, and we think it will be easy to do so.

   ____ We could improve in this area, but we think it will be difficult to do so.

If you found yourself marking the first answer a lot, then you and your partner clearly appreciate the Principle of Long-Term Commitment and have been exploiting that commitment to reinforce each other's efforts to get active and stay active over time.

If your responses tend toward the second answer, then you may not be quite where you want to be, but you are on the right path. Now that you understand how the Principle of Long-Term Commitment affects exercise, you and your partner have a number of great ways to keep each other on track, and there is nothing stopping you from working together to make exercise a permanent part of your lives.

If you found yourself often marking the third answer, then first make sure that you and your partner have a good grasp of the Principle of Long-Term Commitment. Focus intently on the distant horizon, and come together as a couple to articulate what kind of health you envision for yourselves in that time. Remind each other of these vitally important goals, and have the conversations that will motivate you today to be more active, always remembering that getting started is the hardest, and most important, part.

Epilogue

Better Relationships Make
for Healthier Partners . . .
and Healthier Partners Make
for Better Relationships

S O LET'S IMAGINE THAT you and your partner succeed in finding ways to make all these principles work for you—the Principle of Long-Term Influence, the Principle of Mutual Understanding, and the Principle of Mutual Commitment. Your muscles are moving, your hearts are pumping, good food choices are crowding out the bad ones, and you are both feeling the confidence that comes from having an ally by your side. Maybe you are beginning to notice the changes— a spring in your step, a little more energy at the end of the day—and, better still, you know that your healthier habits are registering in your bodies at deep biological levels. Statistically speaking, you are now on track to reduce your risk for a variety of cancers, diabetes, heart failure, stroke, Alzheimer's disease, and osteoporosis—and to live longer lives as a consequence. The "eat right, move more" formula is in effect, enabling you to manage your weight better and achieve greater fitness.

The cells in your bodies are not the only beneficiaries of all your hard work. *As if better health was not a great enough reward by itself, teaming up for a healthier lifestyle produces benefits that extend all the way out to how we think, feel, and behave in our relationships.* All the effort that two people invest in promoting each other's physical health turns out to pay unexpected dividends: teaming up for *personal* fitness increases the chances we will improve our *interpersonal* fitness as well. Partners who collaborate on improving their physical health create three distinct advantages for themselves when it comes to fostering a good relationship—improved psychological health, constructive engagement in the relationship, and a sense of greater contentment and closeness— which in turn contribute to a virtuous cycle that further reinforces all their healthy habits.

Let's look more closely at the three main benefits partners receive as a result of teaming up to improve their physical health:

FIRST, WHEN WE TEAM UP WITH OUR PARTNER TO IMPROVE OUR PHYSICAL HEALTH . . . WE IMPROVE OUR PSYCHOLOGICAL HEALTH AS WELL. How can we best bring out the kindness and understanding that made our partners so attractive in the first place? What steps can any of us take—and what steps can we help our partners to take—to ensure that we are generous and receptive as mates? The evidence is now clear that eating right and moving more work remarkably well at shifting us into precisely those emotional zones that make for better connections:

- Eating right and moving more produce immediate benefits for our mood. While most of us wisely pursue better health for the long-term benefits, plenty of great shorter-term rewards are also apparent. Eating fruits and vegetables increases our level of positive emotion from one day to the next, for example, and physical activity elevates our level of positive emotion for up to three hours after the activity begins.
- Longer-term improvements in our health make us feel more positive and energetic, and less anxious, depressed, and angry. People

who quickly lose large amounts of weight may become anxious and distressed, detracting further from the appeal of diets—while also adding to the difficulty of supporting such dieters. But people who lose five to ten pounds over a twelve-month period experience lower levels of anxiety and depression and higher levels of vitality, self-esteem, and self-control, compared with people who do not lose weight. Switching to a diet that is lower in fats in particular is known to reduce fatigue and feelings of anger and hostility.

- As diet and exercise improve, the quality of our sleep improves as well. Poor sleep wreaks havoc on our mood, our ability to think and concentrate, our inclination to exercise, and even our ability to resist unhealthy snacks. Fortunately, as we get the upper hand on our eating and exercise habits, sleep improves as well. The sleep benefits that come are as likely for men as they are for women, and they are evident in experimental studies of weight-loss programs and in naturalistic studies of weight change.

- Exercise is an especially good way to improve our ability to manage stress. Few of us are at our best when the demands we face are greater than the resources we have available to meet them. But exercise allows us to hit the reset button on stress: people who feel stressed at work often go on to become irritable and depressed, as you would expect, but this effect is reduced sharply among people who exercise regularly—and the reduction grows the more you exercise.

- Being physically active and eating healthier foods makes us mentally sharper. In fact, experiments show that diets high in fat and sugar reduce learning and levels of brain-derived neurotrophic factor (BDNF), a protein that promotes the growth of new neurons in our brains. When we exercise, and when we improve our diets, mental functioning improves—probably because BDNF levels rise as well.

In short, a healthier mate is a happier mate. By encouraging each other to become physically healthier, partners naturally encourage greater psychological health as well. Let's be clear: a vegetable here and a brisk walk there will not have any lasting effect on us or on our relationships. But partners who collaborate to make even small, lasting upgrades in the foods they eat and the calories they burn will be able to approach each other with less stress, less irritability, and more energy.

SECOND, WHEN WE TEAM UP WITH OUR PARTNER TO IMPROVE OUR PHYSICAL HEALTH . . . WE BECOME MORE CONSTRUCTIVELY ENGAGED IN OUR RELATIONSHIP. We are revealing no trade secret in saying that relationships change with the passing of time, and we are betraying no professional confidences by telling you that these changes tend to be for the worse and not the better. But why should it be that relationships, on average, lose their luster as the years pass? Why isn't it the case that, with every passing day, our bonds grow stronger and those great feelings we experienced in the first few months of our relationships grow only deeper and sweeter? The reason, it appears, involves something called self-expansion. In the very early stages of a relationship, our sense of who we are and who we might become expands automatically and without effort, just by being with our new partner. We expand our own identity by taking on the identity and capacities of this person—his or her friends, knowledge, preferences, future prospects, possessions—and all this new growth feels terrific. But nothing this good lasts forever. Whatever substance Cupid puts on his arrows eventually loses potency. As our relationships progress, we become accustomed to who our partners are and what they offer us, and our partners do the same. If we want to continue to gain the benefits that come from expanding and enriching our lives, we need to get on our feet and discover new ways to grow:

- Sharing activities that are new, exciting, arousing, and challenging makes our relationships better. As it turns out, getting on our feet is an ideal way to get started. In one experiment, for example, couples who were assigned to participate in new and exciting activities (hiking, skiing, and dancing, for example) for ninety minutes each week over ten weeks ended up being significantly happier in their relationships, even when compared with people who were assigned to engage in less exciting but pleasant activities (things like visiting friends, going to church, seeing a movie, creative cooking). We also know that couples feel closer right after engaging in exciting activities together. Imagine that! The very same activities that allow us to manage our weight successfully also allow us to keep our relationships fresh and healthy. If you are just getting started on building exercise into your daily schedule, try doing it as a couple, and try to keep challenging yourselves as you move forward. If you prefer to do most of your exercising on your own, find a way to check in on each other's progress, and consider coupling up occasionally to get your hearts pounding in unison.

- Healthier couples have better sex lives. You are already way ahead of us if you are wondering whether one of the hallmarks of a good relationship—a satisfying sex life—improves when partners begin to eat right and move more. The answer is: absolutely. People who report very good or excellent health also report more active and more fulfilling sex lives, and they will remain sexually active for several years longer than their less-healthy peers. Better still, when sedentary men and women in their forties and fifties lose weight and become more fit under controlled conditions, they feel more sexually attractive, get a boost in sexual desire, and are more comfortable with their bodies, compared with people who do not improve their health. In fact, not only does fitness improve virtually every dimension of our sexual functioning, but these benefits often begin quite soon after the program begins, grow larger with greater gains in fitness, and persist even after weight loss stabilizes.

Alas, some bubbles must be burst. The appealing idea that a healthy sex life might be a great way to burn a lot of calories has been unceremoniously dashed recently in the *New England Journal of Medicine*. Dr. Krista Casazza and her colleagues write, "Given that the average bout of sexual activity lasts about 6 minutes, a man in his early to mid-30s might expend approximately 21 calories during sexual intercourse. Of course, he would spend roughly one third that amount of energy just watching television, so the incremental benefit of one bout of sexual activity with respect to energy expended is plausibly on the order of 13 calories." Still, it is a great six minutes, way better than most television, and a great way for partners to stay close—and it is more likely to occur when partners are collaborating to improve their diet and burn calories in other exciting ways.

FINALLY, WHEN WE TEAM UP WITH OUR PARTNER TO IMPROVE OUR PHYSICAL HEALTH . . . WE BECOME CLOSER AND MORE CONTENT IN OUR RELATIONSHIP. There are few better ways to convey the depth of our affection than by noticing, and reaching out to support, the needs and goals of loved ones. We are built to nurture others, but we also are built to respond when others nurture us, and so our relationships naturally grow stronger when both partners demonstrate that the other person's goals and welfare are a high priority. Because we are hardwired for social connection, we get a remarkable boost at those times when we do actively team up and care for each other: we become closer and more content in our relationship.

- Teaming up makes us more cooperative and effective when solving relationship disagreements. Partners who are more effective at teaming up in support of each other's personal goals create a shared platform for discussing *other* key issues in their relationship. Greater connection around personal goals, for example, has been shown to reduce the amount of anger and frustration that partners later express when they work on resolving major disagreements in their relationship. As partners find more and more ways to demonstrate that they are allies and team-mates, conflict subsides and relationships remain strong.

- Teaming up makes us more confident and brings us closer to who we want to be. Attempting to lose ten pounds or get on the treadmill three times per week are important and specific goals on their own, but often they get bundled into bigger visions and aspirations we have for ourselves—like being healthy and fit, staying young and aging well, remaining attractive to our partners, and so on. Research on the Michelangelo phenomenon—so-called because the famous sculptor believed that his task was to reveal the ideal forms that lay dormant in his huge slabs of stone—confirms this idea: partners who team up effectively bring each other closer to their ideal selves. Like a self-fulfilling prophecy, the more partners perceive and treat each other as though they already are en route to becoming their ideal selves, the more they actually go on to achieve those characteristics.

- Teaming up increases the chances we will actually achieve our personal goals. Couples who are observed being more supportive and less critical when discussing their goals for self-improvement are much more likely to achieve those goals over the next twelve months than those who are less supportive and more critical. These benefits are not simply a reflection of how *generally* warm and understanding partners are, or how much individuals *want* to achieve their goals, but they result when partners deliver the kind of support their mates need most. Most of us feel great when we meet our personal goals, and when we recognize that our partners have been instrumental in helping us do so, then both people benefit.

When we think about what makes a relationship strong, our minds turn first to candlelit dinners, heart-to-heart talks about the big issues, a relaxing weekend retreat, self-help books about good communication, a cruise or long vacation, maybe even a visit to a couples counselor when the going gets tough. All are commendable strategies. But what can we do each and every day, day in, day out, throughout the year, to keep our relationship fresh and vital? Our answer is that simple gestures of caring, gestures that are ordinary and invisible but no less affectionate—"*I am going for a walk, will you join me?*" "*I made salads for lunch, do you want some tuna on yours?*" "*How about if I keep an eye on the kids while you go to the gym?*"—have the greatest chance of bringing us closer to our goals for better health and closer to each other as well.

CODA

There is nothing new in the idea that we draw from deep personal connections to promote the health of loved ones. We are built to nurture others, and even when the sacrifices are great, our innate capacity to care shines through. But merely possessing this capacity does not mean we use it as wisely or as well as we might, as we have shown repeatedly throughout this book. In fact, when it comes to two adults striving to team up to eat right and move more every day, mobilizing care and effective support can be difficult. Maybe that's because the immediate need to act is not so obvious, or because our unhealthy habits just become an accepted and intractable part of our lives. Either way, in situations like these, our innate capacity to care needs to be activated and channeled. This is the new idea in *Love Me Slender*—that just by knowing a few key principles, partners are empowered to incorporate proactive, preventive health care into their daily lives. While we all naturally *care about* our partners, locating responsibility for our health squarely within our immediate social circles gives both partners entirely new ways of *caring for* each other. This shift, from the passive *caring about* to the active *caring for,* captures the essence of our message, and it is this shift that comes about when two partners implement our principles on a regular basis.

Is it any wonder that love, arguably the most powerful force in our lives, would emerge as the best hope that any of us have to eat right, move more, and live well?

Acknowledgments

Throughout these pages, we have argued that good health rests on a foundation of good relationships. We have learned that good books rest on the same foundation, and indeed *Love Me Slender* would not exist without the generous and enthusiastic support of a number of wonderful people and organizations.

We thank all the couples who have consented to participate in our research over the years, and whose words provided us with the main idea and the raw material for this book. We are very grateful to these couples for sharing their health-related struggles and successes with us, as it was their honesty and candor that inspired us to find order in all the complexities that arise when two people who love each other try to improve their health behaviors.

The National Institutes of Health provided us with the research funds that we needed to collect the information that we report here. The NIH is a wellspring of support for scientific inquiry in the United States, and we are very fortunate to have access to these resources.

Rob McQuilkin, our literary agent, could not have been more helpful, or more professional, in transforming our initial proposal for this book into a finished product. We were fortunate to have had Rob's astute guidance and insights on every major decision regarding this project, and his patience and kindness never failed to exceed our expectations.

Michelle Howry, our brilliant editor at Simon & Schuster, brought her wealth of experience to bear on every facet and every page of this book. Right from the start Michelle had an intuitive grasp of all that we hoped to accomplish with this project, and thanks to her efforts—and those of her sterling production team—we have done that and more. Special thanks go to Stacy

Creamer, David Falk, Sally Kim, Brendan Culliton, Sophie Vershbow, Ana Paula de Lima, Benjamin Holmes, Beth Maglione, and Ruth Lee-Mui.

We are grateful to Sharbari Kamat, who passed the editorial torch to Michelle Howry; Sharbari's enthusiasm and vision in the early stages of this project gave us the motivation we needed to focus our message and tighten our prose.

Amber Piatt, Davina Simantob, Arielle Ered, Elizabeth Glanzer, and Sravya Mallam, our transcribers, pored over hours of videotapes. Their boundless energy, talent, and insights were instrumental in enabling us to identify the crucial conversations that formed a large part of this book.

David Lederman participated in our early conversations about possible book projects, and played a crucial role in turning us toward the health and wellness of the couples we have been studying.

Attorney Zick Rubin deserves special recognition for connecting us with Rob McQuilkin, and for providing us with sage counsel in all of our book-writing endeavors.

Thomas also acknowledges the generosity and support of his immediate family: Thanks to my parents, Charles and Mary, for underwriting my education, for supporting my career, and for showing me what a healthy and lasting marriage is all about. I also thank my children, Timothy and Nicholas, not for helping me to write this book but for distracting me so well when I was not doing so. Finally, I thank the person I can never thank enough, my wife, friend, colleague, and confidante of more than twenty-five years, Cindy Yee-Bradbury. Thank you, Cindy, for never letting my accomplishments inflate my ego and never allowing my failures to darken my heart. I cherish our life together and the family we have created more than anything else, and I am grateful that you refrained from pointing this out on all those nights I stayed up so late typing away on this manuscript.

Benjamin has several people to thank as well: I thank my parents, Amiram and Perla Karney, for a lifetime of unwavering support for my education and career, and for providing a safe and loving home to this day. I thank Jessica Schulman, for changing the way I think about health and for our ongoing collaboration. I am thankful every day for my children, Daniella and Gabriel, the finest products of that collaboration and my favorite organisms in the history of the universe. Finally, I thank Ali Borden, for insights too numerous and profound to list.

Endnotes

A NOTE ABOUT OUR COUPLES

vii *being young and happy*: J. Sobal, B. Rauschenbach, and E. A. Frongillo, "Marital Status Changes and Body Weight Changes: A US Longitudinal Analysis," *Social Science and Medicine* 56 (2003): 1543–55. N. The and P. Gordon-Larsen, "Entry Into Romantic Partnership is Associated with Obesity," *Obesity* 17 (2009): 1441–47. D. Umberson, H. Liu, J. Mirowsky, and C. Reczek, "Parenthood and Trajectories of Change in Body Weight Over the Life Course," *Social Science and Medicine* 73 (2011): 1323–31.

viii *evidence does suggest*: C. Reczek, "The Promotion of Unhealthy Habits in Gay, Lesbian, and Straight Intimate Partnerships," *Social Science and Medicine* 75 (2012): 1114–21. C. Reczek and D. Umberson, "Gender, Health Behavior, and Intimate Relationships: Lesbian, Gay, and Straight Contexts," *Social Science and Medicine* 74 (2012): 1783–90.

CHAPTER 1: FROM HEALTHY RELATIONSHIPS TO HEALTHY BODIES

3 *a healthier lifestyle* really does *reduce*: R. Estruch, E. Ros, and J. Salas-Salvado, et al., "Primary Prevention of Cardiovascular Disease with a Mediterranean Diet," *New England Journal of Medicine* 368 (2013): 1279–90. T. S. Church, C. P. Earnest, J. S. Skinner, and S. N. Blair, "Effects of Different Doses of Physical Activity on Cardiorespiratory Fitness Among Sedentary, Overweight, or Obese Postmenopausal Women with Elevated Blood Pressure: A Randomized Controlled Trial," *Journal of the American Medical*

Association 297 (2007): 2081–91. D. Mozaffarian, T. Hao, E. B. Rimm, W. C. Willett, and F. Hu, "Changes in Diet and Lifestyle and Long-term Weight Gain in Women and Men," *New England Journal of Medicine* 364 (2011): 2392–404. D. Riebe, B. Blissmer, G. Greene, M. Caldwell, L. Ruggiero, K. M. Stillwell, and C. R. Nigg, "Long-term Maintenance of Exercise and Healthy Eating Behaviors in Overweight Adults," *Preventive Medicine* 40 (2005): 769–78. Look AHEAD Research Group, "Long-term Effects of a Lifestyle Intervention on Weight and Cardiovascular Risk Factors in Individuals with Type 2 Diabetes Mellitus: Four-year Results of the Look AHEAD Trial," *Archives of Internal Medicine* 170 (2010): 1566–75.

3   *Maintaining a healthy weight*: L. H. Kushi, C. Doyle, and M. McCullough, et al., "American Cancer Society Guidelines on Nutrition and Physical Activity for Cancer Prevention," *CA: A Cancer Journal for Clinicians* 62 (2012): 30–67.

4   *We spend more than $6 billion*: C. L. Bish, H. M. Blanck, and M. K. Serdula, et al., "Diet and Physical Activity Behaviors Among Americans Trying to Lose Weight: 2000 Behavioral Risk Factor Surveillance System," *Obesity Research* 13 (2005): 596–607. J. P. Weiner, S. M. Goodwin, and H. Y. Chang, et al., "Impact of Bariatric Surgery on Health Care Costs of Obese Persons: A 6-Year Follow-up of Surgical and Comparison Cohorts Using Health Plan Data," *JAMA Surgery* (2013): 1–8. "US Weight Loss Market Worth 60.9 Billion," http://www.prweb.com/releases/2011/5/prweb8393658.htm, accessed June 21, 2013. "Cost of Weight Loss in America: Many Americans Would Forgo a Job Promotion to Lose 10 Pounds, Reports Nutrisystem Diet Index," http://www.nutrisystemnews.com/2010/08/cost-of-weight-loss-in-america-many-americans-would-forgo-a-job-promotion-to-lose-10-pounds-reports-nutrisystem-diet-index/, accessed June 21, 2013.

4   *more than 85 percent of us*: Y. Wang, M. A. Beydoun, and L. Liang, et al., "Will All Americans Become Overweight or Obese? Estimating the Progression and Cost of the US Obesity Epidemic," *Obesity* 16 (2008): 2323–30.

5   *50 percent of us are almost completely*: C. D. Harris, K. B. Watson, and S. A. Carlson, et al., "Adult Participation in Aerobic and Muscle-Strengthening Physical Activities—United States, 2011," *Morbidity and Mortality Weekly Report* 62 (2013): 326–30. A. S. Go, D. Mozaffarian, and V. L. Roger, et al., "Executive Summary: Heart Disease and Stroke Statistics—2013 Update," *Circulation* 127 (2013): 143–52. D. E. King, A. G. Mainous III, M.

Carnemolla, and C. J. Everett, "Adherence to Healthy Lifestyle Habits in US Adults, 1988–2006," *American Journal of Medicine* 122 (2009): 528–34. D. E. King, A. G. Mainous III, and C. A. Lambourne, "Trends in Dietary Fiber Intake in the United States, 1999–2008," *Journal of the Academy of Nutrition and Dietetics* 112 (2012): 642–48. P. Coxson, N. R. Cook, and M. Joffres, et al., "Mortality Benefits From US Population-wide Reduction in Sodium Consumption: Novelty and Significance Projections From 3 Modeling Approaches," *Hypertension* 61 (2013): 564–70. R. Rosenheck, "Fast Food Consumption and Increased Caloric Intake: A Systematic Review of a Trajectory Toward Weight Gain and Obesity Risk," *Obesity Reviews* 9 (2008): 535–47.

6   *we are not well equipped*: B. M. King, "The Modern Obesity Epidemic: Ancestral Hunter-Gatherers, and the Sensory/Reward Control of Food Intake," *American Psychologist* 68 (2013): 88–96.

7   *To make matters worse*: J. P. Block, S. K. Condon, and K. Kleinman, et al., "Consumers' Estimation of Calorie Content at Fast Food Restaurants: Cross Sectional Observational Study," *British Medical Journal* 346 (2013): 2907. D. Lansky and K. D. Brownell, "Estimates of Food Quantity and Calories: Errors in Self-report Among Obese Patients," *American Journal of Clinical Nutrition* 35 (1982): 727–32.

7   *the rapid pace of modern life*: D. A. Kessler, *The End of Overeating: Taking Control of the Insatiable American Appetite* (New York: Rodale, 2009).

12   *so robust is the link*: J. T. Cacioppo and W. Patrick, *Loneliness: Human Nature and the Need for Social Connection* (New York: W. W. Norton, 2008). J. Barth, S. Schneider, and R. von Känel, "Lack of Social Support in the Etiology and the Prognosis of Coronary Heart Disease: A Systematic Review and Meta-analysis," *Psychosomatic Medicine* 72 (2010): 229–38.

12   *The social connection we get*: J. Holt-Lunstad, T. B. Smith, and J. B. Layton, "Social Relationships and Mortality Risk: A Meta-analytic Review," *PLoS Medicine* 7 (2010): e316. J. S. House, K. R. Landis, and D. Umberson, "Social Relationships and Health," *Science* 241 (1988): 540–45. C. M. Proulx and L. A. Snyder-Rivas, "The Longitudinal Associations Between Marital Happiness, Problems, and Self-rated Health," *Journal of Family Psychology* 27 (2013): 194–202.

12   *husbands and wives are remarkably similar*: A. Di Castelnuovo, G. Quacquaruccio, and M. B. Donati, et al., "Spousal Concordance for Major Coronary Risk Factors: A Systematic Review and Meta-analysis," *American Journal of Epidemiology* 169 (2009): 1–8. D. M. Meyler, J. P. Stimpson, and

M. K. Peek, "Health Concordance Within Couples: A Systematic Review," *Social Science and Medicine* 64 (2007): 2297–310.

13 *when one partner starts spending more time*: A. L. Jurg, W. Wen, and H. L. Li, et al., "Spousal Correlations for Lifestyle Factors and Selected Diseases in Chinese Couples," *Annals of Epidemiology* 16 (2006): 285–91. S. D. Pike, D. A. Wood, A. L. Kinmonth, and S. G. Thompson, "Change in Coronary Risk and Coronary Risk Factor Levels in Couples Following Lifestyle Intervention: The British Family Heart Study," *Archives of Family Medicine* 6 (1997): 354–60.

13 *In one particularly dramatic illustration*: T. A. Falba and J. L. Sindelar, "Spousal Concordance in Health Behavior Change," *Health Services Research* 43 (2008): 96–116.

13 *some medical professionals now recommend*: J. Hippisley-Cox, C. Coupland, and M. Pringle, et al., "Married Couples' Risk of Same Disease: Cross Sectional Study," *British Medical Journal* 325 (2002): 636–40.

14 *psychologists believe that this responsiveness*: C. E. Cutrona, *Social Support in Marriage* (Thousand Oaks, CA: Sage, 1996). K. T. Sullivan and J. Davila, eds., *Support Processes in Intimate Relationships* (New York: Oxford University Press, 2010).

14 *Partners observed talking to each other*: J. P. Gouin, C. S. Carter, and H. Pournajafi-Nazarloo, et al., "Marital Behavior, Oxytocin, Vasopressin, and Wound Healing," *Psychoneuroendocrinology* 35 (2010): 1082–90.

15 *They recover more quickly*: J. C. Coyne, M. J. Rohrbaugh, and V. Shoham, et al., "Prognostic importance of marital quality for survival of congestive heart failure," *American Journal of Cardiology* 88 (2001): 526–29. M. J. Rohrbaugh, M. R. Mehl, and V. Shoham, et al., "Prognostic Significance of Spouse *We* Talk in Couples Coping with Heart Failure," *Journal of Consulting and Clinical Psychology* 76 (2008): 781–89.

15 *When partners are different in their inclinations*: T. B. Hong, M. M. Franks, and R. Gonzalez, et al., "A Dyadic Investigation of Exercise Support Between Cardiac Patients and Their Spouses," *Health Psychology* 24 (2005): 430–34.

15 *People who are trying to eat better*: V. E. Bovbjerg, B. S. McCann, and D. J. Brief, et al., "Spouse Support and Long-term Adherence to Lipid-lowering Diets," *American Journal of Epidemiology* 141 (1995): 451–60.

16 *They tended to lose twice as much*: A. A. Gorin, H. A. Raynor, and J. Fava, et al., "Randomized Controlled Trial of a Comprehensive Home Environment-Focused Weight-Loss Program for Adults," *Health Psychology* 32 (2013): 128–37.

16 *researchers did not have a complete understanding*: D. R. Black, L. J. Gleser, and K. J. Kooyers, "A Meta-analytic Evaluation of Couples Weight-Loss Programs," *Health Psychology* 9 (1990): 330–47. K. Kelsey, J. L. Earp, and B. G. Kirkley, "Is Social Support Beneficial for Dietary Change? A Review of the Literature," *Family and Community Health* 20 (1997): 70–82. N. McLean, S. Griffin, K. Toney, and W. Hardeman, "Family Involvement in Weight Control, Weight Maintenance and Weight-Loss Interventions: A Systematic Review of Randomised Trials," *International Journal of Obesity* 27 (2003): 987–1005. M. R. DiMatteo, "Social Support and Patient Adherence to Medical Treatment: A Meta-Analysis," *Health Psychology* 23 (2004): 207–18. M. W. Verheijden, J. C. Bakx, and C. van Weel, et al., "Role of Social Support in Lifestyle-Focused Weight Management Interventions," *European Journal of Clinical Nutrition* 59 (2005, Suppl. 1): S179–86. L. M. Martire, R. Schulz, and V. S. Helgeson, et al., "Review and Meta-analysis of Couple-Oriented Interventions for Chronic Illness, " *Annals of Behavioral Medicine* 40 (2010): 325–42.

CHAPTER 2: HOW OUR RELATIONSHIPS AFFECT OUR HEALTH

28 *When husbands are placed*: R. Golan, D. Schwarzfuchs, M. J. Stampfer, and I. Shai, "Halo Effect of a Weight-Loss Trial on Spouses: The DIRECT-Spouse Study," *Public Health Nutrition* 13 (2009): 544–49.

30 *But the Principle of Mutual Influence*: J. W. Thibaut and H. H. Kelley, *The Social Psychology of Groups* (New York: Wiley, 1959).

31 *it is the best predictor that has been found*: N. D. Glenn and C. N. Weaver, "The Contribution of Marital Happiness to Global Happiness," *Journal of Marriage and the Family* 43 (1981): 61–68. D. Heller, D. Watson, and R. Ilies, "The Role of Person Versus Situation In Life Satisfaction: A Critical Examination," *Psychological Bulletin* 130 (2004): 574–600.

31 *wives were each placed in an MRI scanner*: J. A. Coan, H. S. Schaefer, and R. J. Davidson, "Lending a Hand: Social Regulation of the Neural Response to Threat," *Psychological Science* 17 (2006): 1032–39.

32 *having family and friends outside the marriage*: M. A. Lieberman, "The Effects of Social Supports on Response to Stress," in L. Goldberger and S. Breznitz, eds., *Handbook of Stress: Theoretical and Clinical Aspects* (New York: Academic Press, 1982): 764–84.

32 *for couples who cannot rely*: J. C. Coyne and A. DeLongis, "Going Beyond Social Support: The Role of Social Relationships in Adaptation," *Journal of Consulting and Clinical Psychology* 5 (1986): 454–60.

32   *the greatest betrayals occur*: B. M. DePaulo, M. E. Ansfield, S. E. Kirkendol, and J. M. Boden, "Serious Lies," *Basic and Applied Social Psychology* 26 (2004), 147–67.

32   *Partners in unhappy relationships*: G. R. Birchler, R. L. Weiss, and J. P. Vincent, "Multimethod Analysis of Social Reinforcement Exchange between Maritally Distressed and Nondistressed Spouse and Stranger Dyads," *Journal of Personality and Social Psychology* 31 (1975): 349–60.

33   *Each partner's experiences*: L. A. Neff and B. R. Karney, "Stress Crossover in Newlywed Marriage: A Longitudinal and Dyadic Perspective," *Journal of Marriage and Family* 69 (2007): 594–607.

34   *partners have a constant impact*: C. F. Bove, J. Sobal, and B. S. Rauschenbach, "Food Choices Among Newly Married Couples: Convergence, Conflict, Individualism, and Projects," *Appetite* 40 (2003): 25–41. C. N. Markey, J. N. Gomel, and P. M. Markey, "Romantic Relationships and Eating Regulation: An Investigation of Partners' Attempts to Control Each Other's Eating Behaviors," *Journal of Health Psychology* 13 (2008): 422–32.

35   *people who are already having trouble*: B. Wansink, *Mindless Eating: Why We Eat More Than We Think* (New York: Bantam, 2006).

35   *people exercise harder*: N. C. Gyurcsik, S. R. Bray, and D. R. Brittain, "Coping with Barriers to Vigorous Physical Activity During Transition to University," *Family and Community Health* 27 (2004): 130. T. G. Plante, L. Coscarelli, and M. Ford, "Does Exercising with Another Enhance the Stress-Reducing Benefits of Exercise?" *International Journal of Stress Management* 8 (2001): 201–13. N. Triplett, "The Dynamogenic Factors in Pacemaking and Competition," *American Journal of Psychology* 9 (1898): 507–33. C. J. Worringhama and D. M. Messicka, "Social Facilitation of Running: An Unobtrusive Study," *Journal of Social Psychology* 121 (1983): 23–29.

38   *our partners are also our most important sources*: P. L. Berger and H. Kellner, "Marriage and the Construction of Reality: An Exercise in the Microsociology of Knowledge," *Diogenes* 46 (1964): 1–24.

39   *when husbands' and wives' opinions*: W. B. Swann, C. De La Ronde, and J. G. Hixon, "Authenticity and Positivity Strivings in Marriage and Courtship," *Journal of Personality and Social Psychology* 66 (1994): 857–69. L. A. Neff and B. R. Karney, "To Know You Is to Love You: The Implications of Global Adoration and Specific Accuracy for Marital Relationships," *Journal of Personality and Social Psychology* 88 (2005): 480–97.

39   *The way our partners understand us*: S. L. Murray, J. G. Holmes, and D. W. Griffin, "The Self-Fulfilling Nature of Positive Illusions in Romantic

Relationships: Love Is Not Blind, But Prescient," *Journal of Personality and Social Psychology* 71 (1996): 1155–80. C. E. Rusbult, E. J. Finkel, and M. Kumashiro, "The Michelangelo Phenomenon," *Current Directions in Psychological Science* 18 (2009): 305–9.

40   *the most effective couple therapies*: A. Christensen and N. S. Jacobson, *Reconcilable Differences* (New York: Guilford, 2002).

41   *those who also understand each other*: L. A. Neff and B. R. Karney, "To Know You Is to Love You: The Implications of Global Adoration and Specific Accuracy for Marital Relationships," *Journal of Personality and Social Psychology* 88 (2005): 480–97.

46   *they are each more willing to forgo*: J. Weiselquist, C. E. Rusbult, C. A. Foster, and C. R. Agnew, "Commitment, Pro-Relationship Behavior, and Trust in Close Relationships," *Journal of Personality and Social Psychology* 77 (1999): 942–66. P. A. M. Van Lange, C. E. Rusbult, S. M. Drigotas, X. B. Arriaga, B. S. Witcher, and C. L. Cox, "Willingness to Sacrifice in Close Relationships," *Journal of Personality and Social Psychology* 72 (1997): 1373–95.

46   *When shown the same photograph*: D. J. Johnson and C. E. Rusbult, "Resisting Temptation: Devaluation of Alternative Partners as a Means of Maintaining Commitment in Close Relationships," *Journal of Personality and Social Psychology* 57 (1989): 967–80.

47   *that initial urge to strike back*: E. J. Finkel, C. E. Rusbult, M. Kumashiro, and P. A. Hannon, "Dealing with Betrayal in Close Relationships: Does Commitment Promote Forgiveness?" *Journal of Personality and Social Psychology* 82 (2002): 956–74.

48   *As the first few pounds*: J. Polivy and C. P. Herman, "If at First You Don't Succeed: False Hopes of Self-Change," *American Psychologist* 57 (2002): 677–89.

49   *self-control remains very hard*: For a thorough review of research supporting this conclusion, see M. R. Lowe, "Self-Regulation of Energy Intake in the Prevention and Treatment of Obesity: Is It Feasible?" *Obesity Research* 11 (2003, Suppl. 1): 44S–59S.

CHAPTER 3: THE BASICS OF HELPING AND BEING HELPED

63   *Even without actually participating*: R. Golan, D. Schwarzfuchs, M. J. Stampfer, and I. Shai, "Halo Effect of a Weight-Loss Trial on Spouses: The DIRECT-Spouse Study," *Public Health Nutrition* 13 (2009): 544–49.

63   *It's almost like getting*: A. A. Gorin, R. R. Wing, and J. L. Fava, et al., "Weight Loss Treatment Influences Untreated Spouses and the Home

Environment: Evidence of the Ripple Effect," *International Journal of Obesity* 32 (2008): 1678–84. M. Sexton, D. Bross, and J. R. Hebel, et al., "Risk-factor Changes in Wives with Husbands at High Risk of Coronary Heart Disease (CHD): The Spin-Off Effect," *Journal of Behavioral Medicine* 10 (1987): 251–61. T. Matsuo, M. K. Kim, and Y. Murotake, et al., "Indirect Lifestyle Intervention Through Wives Improves Metabolic Syndrome Components in Men," *International Journal of Obesity* 34 (2010): 136–45.

65   *the best support is often so small:* N. Bolger and D. Amarel, "Effects of Social Support Visibility on Adjustment to Stress: Experimental Evidence," *Journal of Personality and Social Psychology* 92 (2007): 458–745.

65   *criticism and nagging almost never:* M. Lewis, C. M. McBride, and K. I. Pollak, et al., "Understanding Health Behavior Change Among Couples: An Interdependence and Communal Coping Approach," *Social Science and Medicine* 62 (2006): 1369–80. M. Lewis and R. M. Butterfield, "Social Control in Marital Relationships: Effect of One's Partner on Health Behaviors," *Journal of Applied Social Psychology* 37 (2007): 298–319. A. L. Meltzer, J. K. McNulty, and B. R. Karney, "Social Support and Weight Maintenance in Marriage: The Interactive Effects of Support Seeking, Support Provision, and Gender," *Journal of Family Psychology* 26 (2012): 678–87. S. A. Novak and G. D. Webster, "Spousal Social Control During a Weight Loss Attempt: A Daily Diary Study," *Personal Relationships* 18 (2011): 224–41. J. S. Tucker and J. S. Mueller, "Spouses' Social Control of Health Behaviors: Use and Effectiveness of Special Strategies," *Personality and Social Psychology Bulletin* 26 (2000): 1120–30.

74   *With his influential* transtheoretical model: J. O. Prochaska and C. C. Di-Clemente, *The Transtheoretical Approach: Crossing the Traditional Boundaries of Change* (Homewood, IL: Irwin, 1984).

74   *Applied to eating right:* C. J. Armitage, P. Sheeran, M. Conner, and M. A. Arden, "Stages of Change or Changes of Stage? Predicting Transitions in Transtheoretical Model Stages in Relation to Healthy Food Choice," *Journal of Consulting and Clinical Psychology* 72 (2004): 491–99.

82   *partners who treat each other with more kindness:* M. D. Johnson, C. L. Cohan, and J. Davila, et al., "Problem-Solving Skills and Affective Expressions as Predictors of Change in Marital Satisfaction," *Journal of Consulting and Clinical Psychology* 73 (2005): 15–27. L. A. Pasch and T. N. Bradbury, "Social Support, Conflict, and the Development of Marital

Dysfunction," *Journal of Consulting and Clinical Psychology* 66 (1998): 219–30.

83 *providing clear expectations:* N. C. Overall, G. J. O. Fletcher, J. A. Simpson, and C. G. Sibley, "Regulating Partners in Intimate Relationships: The Costs and Benefits of Different Communication Strategies," *Journal of Personality and Social Psychology* 96 (2009): 620–39. N. C. Overall, G. J. O. Fletcher, and J. A. Simpson, "Helping Each Other Grow: Romantic Partner Support, Self-Improvement, and Relationship Quality," *Personality and Social Psychology Bulletin* 36 (2010): 1496–513. M. M. Oriña, W. Wood, and J. A. Simpson, "Strategies of Influence in Close Relationships," *Journal of Experimental Social Psychology* 38 (2002): 459–72.

CHAPTER 4: EATING RIGHT AND MUTUAL INFLUENCE
98 *restaurant food tends to be much higher:* See C. Stockmyer, "Remember When Mom Wanted You Home for Dinner?" *Nutrition Reviews* 59 (2001): 57–60.

CHAPTER 5: EATING RIGHT AND MUTUAL UNDERSTANDING
139 *Praise and encouragement motivate:* J. S. Tucker and J. S. Mueller, "Spouses' Social Control of Health Behaviors: Use and Effectiveness of Special Strategies," *Personality and Social Psychology Bulletin* 26 (2000): 1120–30. J. S. Tucker and S. L. Anders, "Social Control of Health Behaviors in Marriage," *Journal of Applied Social Psychology* 31 (2001): 467–85. M.A.P. Stephens, K. S. Rook, and M. M. Franks, et al., "Spouses' Use of Social Control to Improve Diabetic Patients' Dietary Adherence," *Families, Systems, & Health* 28 (2010): 199–208.

CHAPTER 6: EATING RIGHT AND LONG-TERM COMMITMENT
160 *Researchers at Stanford University:* C. D. Gardner, A. Kiazand, S. Alhassan, S. Kim, R. S. Stafford, R. R. Balise, H. C. Kraemer, and A. C. King, "Comparison of the Atkins, Zone, Ornish, and LEARN Diets for Change in Weight and Related Risk Factors Among Overweight Premenopausal Women: The A TO Z Weight Loss Study: A Randomized Trial," *JAMA: The Journal of the American Medical Association* 297 (2007): 969–77.
160 *most people who participate:* M. G. Perri and P. R. Fuller, "Success and Failure in the Treatment of Obesity: Where Do We Go From Here?" *Medicine, Exercise, Nutrition, and Health* 4 (1995): 255–72.

160 *The bad news is*: D. Garner and S. Wooley, "Confronting the Failure of Behavioral and Dietary Treatments for Obesity," *Clinical Psychology Review* 11 (1991): 729–80.

160 *more than 80 percent of dieters*: D. W. Swanson and F. A. Dinello, "Follow-up of Patients Starved for Obesity," *Psychosomatic Medicine* 32 (1970): 209–14.

160 *When it comes to eating habits*: T. Mann, A. J. Tomiyama, E. Westling, A. M. Lew, B. Samuels, and J. Chatman, "Medicare's Search for Effective Obesity Treatments: Diets Are Not the Answer," *American Psychologist* 62 (2007): 220–33.

161 *they are the ones who were able*: S. N. Shick, R. R. Wing, M. L. Klem, M. T. McGuire, J. O. Hill, and H. M. Seagle, "Persons Successful at Long-Term Weight Loss and Maintenance Continue to Consume a Low Calorie, Low Fat Diet," *Journal of the American Dietetic Association* 98 (1998): 408–13.

161 *we are much more likely to sustain*: E. T. Higgins, "Beyond Pleasure and Pain," *American Psychologist* 52 (1997): 1280–1300.

161–62 *when people keep their long-term goals*: G. Oettingen, H. Pak, and K. Schnetter, "Self-Regulation of Goal-Setting: Turning Free Fantasies about the Future into Binding Goals," *Journal of Personality and Social Psychology* 80 (2001): 736.

162 *When we do the same thing*: M. A. Adriaanse, G. Oettingen, P. M. Gollwitzer, E. P. Hennes, D. T. D. de Ridder, and J. B. F. de Wit, "When Planning Is Not Enough: Fighting Unhealthy Snacking Habits by Mental Contrasting with Implementation Intentions (MCII)," *European Journal of Social Psychology* 40 (2010): 1277–93.

169 *we are more likely to persist*: D. Ariely, *The Upside of Irrationality* (New York: HarperCollins, 2010).

170 *their desires are disconnected*: J. Polivy and C. P. Herman, "If at First You Don't Succeed: False Hopes of Self-Change," *American Psychologist* 57 (2002): 677–89.

173 *it happens whenever daydreaming about reaching*: P. M. Gollwitzer and G. Oettingen, "The Emergence and Implementation of Health Goals," *Psychology & Health* 13 (1998): 687–715.

CHAPTER 7: MOVING MORE AND MUTUAL INFLUENCE

195 *one review calculated*: C. D. Reimers, G. Knapp, and A. K. Reimers, "Does Physical Activity Increase Life Expectancy? A Review of the Literature," *Journal of Aging Research* 1–9 (2012).

195 *Older adults who get regular exercise:* W. J. Rejeski and S. L. Mihalko, "Physical Activity and Quality of Life in Older Adults," *The Journals of Gerontology Series A: Biological Sciences and Medical Sciences* 56 (2001, Suppl. 2): 23–35.

195 *even healthy young people:* J. P. Maher, S. E. Doerksen, S. Elavsky, A. L. Hyde, A. L. Pincus, N. Ram, and D. E. Conroy, "A Daily Analysis of Physical Activity and Satisfaction with Life in Emerging Adults," *Health Psychology* 32 (2012): 647–56.

195 *exercise is now being prescribed:* A. Rozanski, "Exercise as Medical Treatment for Depression," *Journal of the American College of Cardiology* 60 (2012): 1064–66.

195 *it has proven to be as effective:* J. A. Blumenthal, A. Sherwood, and M. A. Babyak, et al., "Exercise and Pharmacological Treatment of Depressive Symptoms in Patients with Coronary Heart Disease," *Journal of the American College of Cardiology* 60 (2012): 1053–63.

195 *exercise is not quite as effective:* C. J. Zelasko, "Exercise for Weight Loss," *Journal of the American Dietetic Association* 95 (1995): 1414–17.

195 *programs focusing on diet plus exercise:* W. C. Miller, D. Koceja, and E. Hamilton, "A Meta-Analysis of the Past 25 Years of Weight Loss Research Using Diet, Exercise or Diet Plus Exercise Intervention," *International Journal of Obesity* 21 (1997): 941–47.

196 *one representative set of guidelines:* S. N. Blair, M. J. LaMonte, and M. Z. Nichaman, "The Evolution of Physical Activity Recommendations: How Much Is Enough?" *The American Journal of Clinical Nutrition* 79 (2004): 913S–20S.

196 *the Surgeon General of the United States concluded:* US Department of Health and Human Services, *The Surgeon General's Vision for a Healthy and Fit Nation* (Rockville, MD: US Department of Health and Human Services, Office of the Surgeon General, 2010).

196 *less than half of adults:* Centers for Disease Control and Prevention, *State Indicator Report on Physical Activity* (Atlanta, GA: US Department of Health and Human Services, 2010).

200 *Exercise programs are indeed more effective:* P. Gellert, J. P. Ziegelmann, L. M. Warner, and R. Schwarzer, "Physical Activity Intervention in Older Adults: Does a Participating Partner Make a Difference?" *European Journal of Ageing* 8 (2011): 211–19.

212 *This is called reward substitution:* D. Ariely, *The Upside of Irrationality* (New York: HarperCollins, 2010).

CHAPTER 8: MOVING MORE AND MUTUAL UNDERSTANDING

231 *When partners are at different stages*: M. M. Franks, C. G. Shields, and E. Lim, et al., "I Will if You Will: Similarity in Married Partners' Readiness to Change Health Risk Behaviors," *Health Education and Behavior* 39 (2012): 324–31.

242 *when we are anxious and vulnerable*: S. L. Murray, J. G. Holmes, and D. W. Griffin, et al., "The Mismeasure of Love: How Self-doubt Contaminates Relationship Beliefs," *Personality and Social Psychology Bulletin* 27 (2001): 423–36.

243 *anticipating problems and engaging*: G. Stadler, G. Oettingen, and P. Gollwitzer, "Physical Activity in Women: Effects of a Self-Regulation Intervention," *American Journal of Preventive Medicine* 36 (2009): 29–34.

CHAPTER 9: MOVING MORE AND LONG-TERM COMMITMENT

256 *42 percent of children*: R. P. Troiano, D. Berrigan, K. W. Dodd, L. C. Mâsse, T. Tilert, and M. McDowell, "Physical Activity in the United States Measured by Accelerometer," *Medicine and Science in Sports and Exercise* 40 (2008): 181–88.

256 *physical activity continues to decline*: R. M. Malina, "Physical Activity and Fitness: Pathways from Childhood to Adulthood," *American Journal of Human Biology* 13 (2001): 162–72. D. P. Scharff, S. Homan, M. Kreuter, and L. Brennan, "Factors Associated with Physical Activity in Women Across the Life Span: Implications for Program Development," *Women & Health* 29 (1999): 115–34.

256 *busier schedules, competing obligations*: P. Gordon-Larsen, M. C. Nelson, and B. M. Popkin, "Longitudinal Physical Activity and Sedentary Behavior Trends," *American Journal of Preventive Medicine* 27 (2004): 277–83.

256 *By junior high school*: T. M. DiLorenzo, R. C. Stucky-Ropp, J. S. Vander Wal, and H. J. Gotham, "Determinants of Exercise among Children. II. A Longitudinal Analysis," *Preventive Medicine* 27 (1998): 470–77.

256 *And the battle just heats up*: J. Lefevre, R. M. Philippaerts, and K. Delvaux, et al., "Daily Physical Activity and Physical Fitness From Adolescence to Adulthood: A Longitudinal Study," *American Journal of Human Biology* 12 (2000): 487–97.

257 *they are even less physically active*: M. L. Booth, A. Bauman, N. Owen, and C. J. Gore, "Physical Activity Preferences, Preferred Sources of Assistance, and Perceived Barriers to Increased Activity among Physically Inactive Australians," *Preventive Medicine* 26 (1997): 131–37.

257 *Older adults, in contrast*: D. P. Scharff, S. Homan, M. Kreuter, and L. Brennan, "Factors Associated with Physical Activity in Women Across the Life Span: Implications for Program Development," *Women & Health* 29 (1999): 115–34.

257 *there is evidence that over time*: D. E. Conroy, J. P. Maher, S. Elavsky, A. L. Hyde, and S. E. Doerksen, "Sedentary Behavior as a Daily Process Regulated by Habits and Intentions," *Health Psychology* (2013).

262 *even advantaged partners are less satisfied*: N. W. Van Yperen and B. P. Buunk, "A Longitudinal Study of Equity and Satisfaction in Intimate Relationships," *European Journal of Social Psychology* 20 (1990): 287–309.

265 *When working out is uncomfortable*: D. M. Williams, S. Dunsiger, J. T. Ciccolo, and B. A. Lewis, et al., "Acute Affective Response to a Moderate-Intensity Exercise Stimulus Predicts Physical Activity Participation 6 and 12 Months Later," *Psychology of Sport and Exercise* 9 (2008): 231–45.

266 *when people choose their own level*: P. Ekkekakis, "Let Them Roam Free?: Physiological and Psychological Evidence for the Potential of Self-Selected Exercise Intensity in Public Health," *Sports Medicine* 39 (2009): 857–88. P. Ekkekakis, G. Parfitt, and S. J. Petruzzello, "The Pleasure and Displeasure People Feel when They Exercise at Different Intensities: Decennial Update and Progress Towards a Tripartite Rationale for Exercise Intensity Prescription," *Sports Medicine* 41 (2011): 641–71.

267 *Psychologists have coined the term*: L. Y. Abramson, M. E. P. Seligman, and J. F. Teasdale, "Learned Helplessness in Humans: Critique and Reformulation," *Journal of Abnormal Psychology* 87 (1978): 49–74.

267 *Caregivers who experience burnout*: M. C. Angermeyer, N. Bull, S. Bernert, S. Dietrich, and A. Kopf, "Burnout of Caregivers: A Comparison Between Partners of Psychiatric Patients and Nurses," *Archives of Psychiatric Nursing* 20 (2006): 158–65.

EPILOGUE: BETTER RELATIONSHIPS MAKE FOR
HEALTHIER PARTNERS . . . AND HEALTHIER PARTNERS
MAKE FOR BETTER RELATIONSHIPS

275 *you are now on track to reduce*: L. Djoussé, J. A. Driver, and J. M. Gaziano, "Relation Between Modifiable Lifestyle Factors and Lifetime Risk of Heart Failure," *Journal of the American Medical Association* 302 (2009): 394–400. E. S. Ford, M. M. Bergmann, and J. Kroger, et al., "Healthy Living Is the Best Revenge: Findings from the European Prospective Investigation into Cancer and Nutrition—Potsdam Study," *Archives of Internal Medicine* 169

(2009): 1355–62. Y. Gu, J. W. Nieves, and Y. Stern, et al., "Diet and Prevention of Alzheimer Disease," *Archives of Neurology* 67 (2010): 699–706. D. E. King, A. G. Mainous, and M. E. Geesey, "Turning Back the Clock: Adopting a Healthy Lifestyle in Middle Age," *American Journal of Medicine* 120 (2007): 598–603. L. H. Kushi, et al., "American Cancer Society Guidelines on Nutrition and Physical Activity for Cancer Prevention: Reducing the Risk of Cancer With Healthy Food Choices and Physical Activity, *Cancer Journal for Clinicians* 62 (2012): 30–67. A. Nicolucci, S. Balducci, and P. Cardelli, et al., "Relationship of Exercise Volume to Improvements of Quality of Life with Supervised Exercise Training in Patients with Type 2 Diabetes in a Randomized Controlled Trial: The Italian Diabetes and Exercise Study (IDES)," *Diabetologia* 55 (2012): 579–88. D. E. R. Warburton, C. W. Nicol, and S. S. D. Bredin, "Health Benefits of Physical Exercise: The Evidence," *Canadian Medical Association Journal* 174 (2006): 801–9.

275 *The "eat right, move more" formula*: D. Mozaffarian, T. Hao, and E. B. Rimm, et al., "Changes in Diet and Lifestyle and Long-Term Weight Gain in Women and Men," *The New England Journal of Medicine* 364 (2011): 2392–404. D. Riebe, B. Blissmer, and G. Greene, et al., "Long-Term Maintenance of Exercise and Healthy Eating Behaviors in Overweight Adults," *Preventive Medicine* 40 (2005): 769–78. Look AHEAD Research Group, "Long-Term Effects of a Lifestyle Intervention on Weight and Cardiovascular Risk Factors in Individuals with Type 2 Diabetes Mellitus: Four-Year Results of the Look AHEAD Trial," *Archives of Internal Medicine* 170 (2010): 1566–75.

276 *Eating fruits and vegetables*: B. A. White, C. C. Horwath, and T. S. Conner, "Many Apples a Day Keep the Blues Away—Experiences of Negative and Positive Affect and Food Consumption in Young Adults," *British Journal of Health Psychology* (2013). M. Wichers, F. Peeters, and B. P. F. Rutten, et al., "A Time-Lagged Momentary Assessment of Daily Life Physical Activity and Affect," *Health Psychology* 31 (2012): 135–44.

277 *Switching to a diet that is lower in fats*: G. D. Brinkworth, J. D. Buckley, and M. Noakes, et al., "Long-Term Effects of a Very Low-Carbohydrate Diet and a Low-Fat Diet On Mood and Cognitive and Function," *Archives of Internal Medicine* 169 (2009): 1873–80. J.-P. Chaput, V. Drapeau, and M. Hetherington, et al., "Psychobiological Impact of a Progressive Weight Loss Program in Obese Men," *Physiology and Behavior* 86 (2005): 224–32. C. Swencionis, J. Wylie-Rosett, and M. Lent, et al., "Weight Change, Psychological Well-Being, and Vitality in Adults Participating in a

Cognitive-Behavioral Weight Loss Program," *Health Psychology* 32 (2013): 439–46.

277 *The sleep benefits that come*: A. Anandam, M. Akinusi, and T. Kufel, et al., "Effects of Dietary Weight Loss on Obstructive Sleep Apnea: A Meta-Analysis," *Sleep and Breathing* 17 (2012): 227–34. P. E. Peppard, T. Young, and M. Palta, et al., "Longitudinal Study of Moderate Weight Change and Sleep-Disordered Breathing," *Journal of the American Medical Association* 284 (2000): 3015–21. K. Peuhkuri, N. Shivola, and R. Korpela, "Diet Promotes Sleep Duration and Quality," *Nutrition Research* 32 (2012): 309–19.

277 *people who feel stressed at work*: P. Salmon, "Effects of Physical Exercise on Anxiety, Depression, and Sensitivity to Stress: A Unifying Theory," *Clinical Psychology Review* 21 (2001): 33–61. S. Toker and M. Biron, "Job Burnout and Depression: Unraveling Their Temporal Relationship and Considering the Role of Physical Activity," *Journal of Applied Psychology* 97 (2012): 699–710. A. Tsatsoulis and S. Fountoulakis, "The Protective Role of Exercise on Stress System Dysregulation and Comorbidities," *Annals of the New York Academy of Sciences* 1083 (2006): 196–213.

277 *When we exercise, and when we improve*: H. Francis and R. Stevenson, "The Longer-Term Impacts of Western Diet on Human Cognition and the Brain," *Appetite* 63 (2013): 119–28. F. B. Gillison, S. M. Skevington, and A. Sato, et al., "The Effects of Exercise On Quality of Life in Clinical and Healthy Populations: A Meta-Analysis," *Social Science and Medicine* 68 (2009): 1700–10. C. H. Hillman, K. I. Erickson, and A. F. Kramer, "Be Smart, Exercise Your Heart: Exercise Effects on Brain and Cognition," *Nature Reviews Neuroscience* 9 (2008): 58–65. R. Molteni, A. Wu, and S. Vaynman, et al., "Exercises Reverses the Harmful Effects of Consumption of a High-Fat Diet on Synaptic and Behavioral Plasticity Associated to the Action of Brain-Derived Neurotrophic Factor," *Neuroscience* 123 (2004): 429–40.

278 *We are revealing no trade secret*: T. L. Huston and A. L. Vangelisti, "Socioemotional Behavior and Satisfaction in Marital Relationships: A Longitudinal Study," *Journal of Personality and Social Psychology* 61 (1991): 721–33.

278 *we need to get on our feet*: A. Aron, C. C. Norman, and E. N. Aron, et al., "Couples' Shared Participation in Novel and Arousing Activities and Experienced Relationship Quality," *Journal of Personality and Social Psychology* 78 (2000): 273–84.

278 *couples who were assigned to participate*: C. Reissman, A. Aron, and M. R. Bergen, "Shared Activities and Marital Satisfaction: Causal Direction and

Self-Expansion Versus Boredom," *Journal of Social and Personal Relationships* 10 (1993): 243–54.

279 *couples feel closer right after engaging*: J. M. Graham, "Self-Expansion and Flow in Couples' Momentary Experiences: An Experience Sampling Study," *Journal of Personality and Social Psychology* 95 (2008): 679–94.

279 *one of the hallmarks of a good relationship*: E. Lawrence, et al., "Objective Ratings of Relationship Skills Across Multiple Domains as Predictors of Marital Satisfaction Trajectories," *Journal of Social and Personal Relationships* 25 (2008): 445–66.

279 *People who report very good or excellent health*: S. T. Lindau and N. Gavrilova, "Sex, Health, and Years of Sexually Active Life Gained Due to Good Health: Evidence from Two US Population-Based Cross-Sectional Surveys of Ageing," *British Medical Journal* 340 (2010): c810.

279 *these benefits often begin quite soon*: B. P. Gupta, H. Murad, and M. M. Clifton, et al., "The Effect of Lifestyle Modification and Cardiovascular Risk Factor Reduction on Erectile Dysfunction: A Systematic Review and Meta-Analysis," *Archives of Internal Medicine* 171 (2011): 1797–803. R. L. Kolotkin, M. Binks, and R. D. Crosby, et al., "Improvements in Sexual Quality of Life after Moderate Weight Loss," *International Journal of Impotence* 20 (2008): 487–92. R. L. Kolotkin, C. Zunker, and T. Østbye, "Sexual Functioning and Obesity," *Obesity* 20 (2012): 2325–38. J. R. White, D. A. Case, D. McWhirter, and A. M. Mattison, "Enhanced Sexual Behavior in Exercising Men," *Archives of Sexual Behavior* 19 (1990): 193–209.

280 *the incremental benefit of one bout*: K. Casazza, et al., "Myths, Presumptions, and Facts about Obesity," *New England Journal of Medicine* 368 (2013): 446–54.

281 *As partners find more and more ways*: L. A. Pasch and T. N. Bradbury, "Social Support, Conflict, and the Development of Marital Dysfunction," *Journal of Consulting and Clinical Psychology* 66 (1998): 219–30. K. T. Sullivan, L. A. Pasch, M. D. Johnson, and T. N. Bradbury, "Social Support, Problem-Solving, and the Longitudinal Course of Newlywed Marriage," *Journal of Personality and Social Psychology* 98 (2010): 631–44. J. C. Brunstein, G. Dangelmeyer, and O. C. Schultheiss, "Personal Goals and Social Support in Close Relationships: Effects on Relationship Mood and Marital Satisfaction," *Journal of Personality and Social Psychology* 71 (1996): 1006–19.

281 *the more partners perceive and treat each other*: D. C. Molden, G. M. Lucas, and E. J. Finkel, et al., "Perceived Support for Promotion-Focused and Prevention-Focused Goals: Associations with Well-being in Unmarried

and Married Couples," *Psychological Science* 20 (2009): 787–93. C. E. Rusbult, E. J. Finkel, and M. Kumashiro, "The Michelangelo Phenomenon," *Current Directions in Psychological Science* 18 (2009): 305–9.

281 *Most of us feel great:* J. Gere, U. Schimmack, R. T. Pinkus, and P. Lockwood, "The Effects of Romantic Partners' Goal Congruence on Affective Well-being," *Journal of Research in Personality* 45 (2011): 549–59. N. C. Overall, G. J. O. Fletcher, and J. A. Simpson, "Helping Each Other Grow: Romantic Partner Support, Self-Improvement, and Relationship Quality," *Personality and Social Psychology Bulletin* 36 (2010): 1496–513. L. L. Verhofstadt, A. Buysse, and W. Ickes, et al., "Support Provision in Marriage: The Role of Emotional Similarity and Empathic Accuracy," *Emotion* 8 (2008): 792–802.

282 *We are built to nurture others:* S. E. Taylor, *The Tending Instinct: How Nurturing Is Essential to Who We Are and How We Live* (New York: Henry Holt, 2002).

Index

306 Index

Index 319

mutual understanding and, 129, 138
support and, 10, 67, 93
tensions, 19
diet and, 123, 150, 172–73
exercise and, 190, 199–200, 260
long-term commitment and, 47, 172–73, 260
mutual influence and, 123, 190, 199–200
mutual understanding and, 41, 52, 150
thoughts, thinking, 49
diet and, 97, 102, 105, 132–33, 137, 147, 149–50, 161–62, 171, 176
exercise and, 206, 238, 252, 259–61, 264, 269, 272, 277
long-term commitment and, 46–47, 50, 53, 161–62, 171, 176, 259–61, 264, 269, 272
mutual influence and, 29, 52, 59, 102, 105, 206
mutual understanding and, 38, 41, 73, 76, 132–33, 137, 147, 149–50, 238
support and, 60–61, 73, 76
threats:
exercise and, 208, 224–25, 227–28, 230–35, 244, 259, 269
long-term commitment and, 46, 166, 171, 175, 259, 269
mutual influence and, 31–32, 208
tomatoes, 133, 136
transtheoretical model, 74–75
treadmills, 48, 72, 199, 209, 212, 234

understanding, *see* Mutual Understanding, Principle of

vegetables, 3–5, 58, 210, 235, 276, 278
long-term commitment and, 47–48, 169, 176–77
mutual influence and, 106, 108–9, 116
mutual understanding and, 133–34, 136, 138, 141–42, 146, 148, 235
vegetarian diets, 34, 155, 175
vulnerabilities, 18
mutual influence and, 65, 67
mutual understanding and, 150, 227, 233, 242
support and, 55, 65, 67

Waffler, 225
diet and, 125, 140–51
your partner as, 146–50
waistlines, 13, 37, 155
fat around, 4, 12, 103
walking, 3, 145, 196–97, 266
and benefits of partnerships, 278, 282

and connection between health and relationships, 12–13
mutual influence and, 30, 34, 36–37, 66–67, 190–93, 199, 202–3, 205–6, 209, 212–13, 215
mutual understanding and, 235–36
and unhappiness with weight, 20–22, 24–25
Wansink, Brian, 35
weight, vii, 5, 12, 17, 247, 275, 279
health and, 20, 22, 24–25, 36–37, 40–41, 43, 47, 50–52, 95
management of, 3, 24, 37, 40, 43, 47, 50–52, 150, 156, 195, 235
mutual influence and, 33, 36–37, 101
mutual understanding and, 40–43, 52, 71, 75
support and, 10, 71, 75
unhappiness with, 19–26
weight gain, 8, 24, 41
diet and, 97–98, 114, 126, 128, 133, 149–50, 155–56, 158, 160, 165, 172–74
exercise and, 19–26, 189, 219, 230, 237, 241, 249, 252, 267
in pregnancy, 50–51
support and, 19, 61–62, 85–86
weight lifting, 196, 202, 233, 236, 241
weight loss, 6, 8
and benefits of partnerships, 279–81
diet and, 98–99, 101–3, 109–11, 116, 123, 125–31, 133–37, 141, 146, 151, 155–56, 159–61, 163–72, 177–81, 183–84, 195–96, 215, 264, 277
exercise and, 19–26, 178, 190–92, 194–96, 203–4, 207, 215, 219–20, 222–23, 230–32, 239–40, 248–49
goals for, 10, 50, 98–99, 171, 184
long-term commitment and, 48, 50–51, 84, 161, 163–72, 177–81, 183–84
mutual influence and, 37, 63, 66, 101–3, 109–11, 116, 190–92, 194, 203–4, 207, 215
mutual understanding and, 41, 50, 70, 79, 123, 125–31, 133–37, 141, 146, 151, 230–32, 239–40
partner in seeing it as now or never, 166–70
and Sara and Brian case, 19–26
statistics on, 4–5
support and, 15–16, 18–19, 27, 57, 63, 66, 70, 79, 83–84, 146
sustaining of, 15–16, 159, 161, 165, 182–83, 195–96, 215, 248
timing of, 163–65, 171
Weight Watchers, 79, 135, 181
willpower, 6, 9–10, 19, 48, 99, 176

yogurt, 64, 88, 169

About the Authors

THOMAS N. BRADBURY earned a BA in psychobiology from Hamilton College and a PhD in clinical psychology from the University of Illinois. A Professor of Psychology at the University of California, Los Angeles, since 1990, Dr. Bradbury has received awards for teaching, mentoring, and research, including the Distinguished Early Career Award in 1998 from the American Psychological Association and an honorary academic degree, the *Laurea Honoris Causa*, in 2013 from Università Cattolica del Sacro Cuore in Milan, Italy.

BENJAMIN R. KARNEY earned a BA in psychology from Harvard University and a PhD in social psychology from the University of California, Los Angeles. An award-winning teacher and scholar, Dr. Karney was recognized as the Teacher of the Year in 2003 at the University of Florida, and he received the Early Career Achievement Award in 1996 from the International Network on Personal Relationships. A Professor of Psychology at UCLA since 2007, Dr. Karney was awarded his department's Distinguished Teaching Award in 2011, and twice he has received the Reuben Hill Research and Theory Award for Outstanding Contributions to Family Science from the National Council on Family Relations.

For more than twenty years, Drs. Bradbury and Karney have studied the ways that partners communicate, support each other, and maintain their relationships. Together they founded and codirect the Relationship Institute at UCLA, a center dedicated to engaging the general public with lectures, seminars, and workshops on new discoveries in the field of relationship science (visit their website at www.uclarelationshipinstitute.org).